Fighting Free Radicals

The New Zealand Pine Bark Extract Story

Thorsons

Thorsons
An Imprint of HarperCollins *Publishers*
77–85 Fulham Palace Road,
Hammersmith, London W6 8JB
1160 Battery Street,
San Francisco, California 94111–1213

Published by Thorsons 1998

1 3 5 7 9 10 8 6 4 2

UK Edition

ISBN 0-583-34184-5

ENZOGENOL™ is the Registered Trademark of ENZO Nutraceuticals Ltd,
P O Box 1770, Christchurch, New Zealand.

"The main purpose of this book is to provide information.
It is not intended to be substituted for medical advice.
Please consult your health professional if the need for one is required."

New Zealand Edition
Published by
The Pacific Scientific Press
Christchurch   Auckland

Contents

Introduction

This book sets out to explain in terms as simple as possible why, how and with what results free radicals attack our bodies, and how antioxidants form the first line of defence against them. As you are probably well aware, the subject of free radicals and antioxidants is extremely complex. This book should fill some gaps in your knowledge and offer much fascinating background which will make it easier for you to explain to your friends, neighbours and relatives why you are taking a compound made from the bark of *Pinus radiata*. This species has flourished in New Zealand where it is the predominant sustainable forestry plantation species; some readers may be more familiar with it as Monterey pine, the name denoting its provenance, the Monterey Peninsula on the Pacific coast of the United States.

This book is structured somewhat unconventionally in that it summarises the whole story in Chapter 1. The conclusion is so good, how could we possibly leave it until the end? Most books written on the subject recently, and there have been more than an armful, take the reader through a tortuous labyrinth of biochemistry in order to support the logic of the wonderful ending. The reader versed in chemistry will find some of that material in this book also. The origins and behaviour of free radicals are well described in Chapter 5. If it is too detailed for your own grasp of matters chemical, skip over it; it is not essential to grasp the biochemistry fully to understand the enormity of the benefits that antioxidants can confer on health. You are still assured of a good read, and a veritable gold-mine of fascinating information on your body and your health.

If you already know the basic story of free radicals and antioxidants, and are more interested in greater technical detail and in the uniqueness of Enzogenol, you could skip Chapter 1 but bear in mind that it will be most helpful in introducing others to the subject.

About the Authors

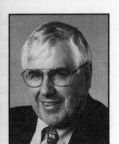

Kelvin Duncan, B.Sc.(Hons.), Ph.D., MRNZSS, NYAS, Dip. Statistics.

Dr Duncan is the Dean of Science at the University of Canterbury. He is a renowned biologist and is the avid chaser of "Red Queens", the biological interactions of organisms at biochemical and physiological level, focusing on augmenting human defence mechanisms. He has worked with and developed many bioactive compounds of human interest. He holds a number of patents and is an expert on managing toxicity trials. He is an advisor to a number of countries in Europe, South East Asia, Latin America and the Pacific Islands.

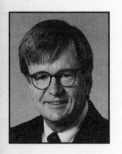

Larry Stenswick, M.A.

Mr Stenswick has served the New Zealand and United States governments in senior international trade positions. He has also headed a number of very successful commercial enterprises engaged in the production, processing and distribution of natural food products, where he consistently championed innovative science-based development. He is a special advisor to several leading international nutraceutical companies.

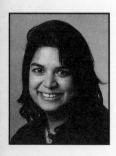

Joshna Dayal, B.E.(Hons)

Ms Dayal is a chemical and process engineer, and a specialist in the field of natural product processing. She has extensive experience in product and process development, and has managed several substantial and innovative projects from conception through laboratory-scale development to full-scale commercial production.

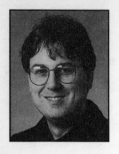

Steven Gieseg, B.Sc. (Hons), Ph.D.

Dr Gieseg lectures in animal and free radical biochemistry at the University of Canterbury. He also has a small research team of post-graduate students studying free radical-mediated processes and antioxidant protection mechanisms. He has been a member of the International Free Radical Society since 1990 and is the South Island representative of the Australasian Free Radical Society.

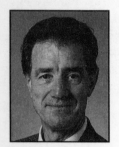

Ian Gilmour, M.E., C.Eng., M.I.Chem.E.

Mr Gilmour is a senior lecturer in chemical and process engineering at the University of Canterbury with years of experience in developing extraction processes for natural products, including the harnessing of microbial and fungal cultures for biological treatment of waste. He has a special interest in developing environmentally-friendly technologies for converting waste into valuable products.

Chapter 1

The Pine Bark Story
New Zealands Own Pine Bark Extract

New Zealand Pine Bark is a new powerful antioxidant derived from the bark of selected *Pinus radiata*. As this chapter – and Chapter 7 in greater detail – will explain, pine bark has recently been established as containing the most comprehensive complex of natural antioxidants yet discovered. Groundbreaking processing technology has made it possible to combine all of those antioxidants in a capsule in exactly the same ratios as are present in the bark of the tree. This revolutionary process, trade marked as Enzogenol, now has a patent pending creating *not only a unique, but also the most complete and valuable antioxidant supplement that it has yet been possible to create.* But, firstly, let's go back to the beginning ....

Oxidation and Antioxidants

Antioxidants are biochemical entities which, as their name suggests, prevent oxidation. Antioxidants are marvellous things, useful in all kinds of situations where we don't want oxidation to occur.

In the third form science sense, oxidation is a process which sees oxygen binding to other elements or compounds to form oxides. The most widely understood example would be the oxidation of hydrogen atoms to create water. Oxidation happens everywhere, all the time, because oxygen is everywhere – in the air and in almost every living thing. Everywhere we look we can see oxidation in progress. Iron rusts because it is being oxidised. The flesh of an apple cut open or bitten into goes brown quite quickly as a result of oxidation. Paint dries because of oxidation.

Oxidation happens inside our bodies, too. Even as you read this book, the last meal you ate is being oxidised in your body's tissues. Oxidation is an essential process in the life cycle of every living organism. But the old adage holds true: too much of a good thing can be bad for you. If left uncontrolled, oxygen would just carry on and oxidise your body to death. Your body 'knows' this, so it produces and maintains an and maintains an army of oxygen police, called antioxidants. Antioxidants also occur elsewhere in nature, as we shall see later, so those generated within the human body are differentiated by the term 'endogenous' antioxidants.

The most commonly discussed of these is an enzyme called superoxide dismutase which attacks the very prominent oxidising free radical, superoxide. The discovery of this enzyme, in fact, was one of the turning points in the acceptance by mainstream science of the free radical theory of damage and disease. It appeared then, and still does, to have no other function than to neutralise superoxide. Vitamins C and E are also antioxidants, which sheds more light on why so many claims have been made for their efficacy over the years. Indeed, as we will see, a good deal of the emerging information on antioxidants and free radicals is making sense of a tremendous amount of conventional, and even traditional, thinking about diet and health.

To see how antioxidants operate, we need to know a little about the oxygen species they are designed to control. Before we go too much further, let's ease up a little on oxygen *per se*. Over the years, scientists have come to use the term 'oxidation' for the action of free radicals of any element. Oxidation, then, can be a reaction from which oxygen is absent but which involve free radicals of one kind or another.

Our bodies are, among other things, a mass of millions of chemical reactions involving oxidations taking place every second. Things are very, very busy in there! All chemical reactions, including those digesting your dinner, involve atoms or molecules binding onto other atoms or molecules to form new substances. Sometimes, however, you can't write a neat and tidy equation for every one of those reactions, as in many cases the newly formed substance doesn't use up all the constituents of the reaction. Little spare bits fly off with minds of their own. A quick revision of basic chemistry is perhaps appropriate: atoms consist of pairs of electrons orbiting a nucleus containing protons and neutrons. Now, these little spare bits flying off the reactions mentioned above are often half-baked; they are atoms with single or 'unpaired' electrons in their orbits. Naturally, they are inclined to rectify this situation quickly so they rush around seeking something from which they can rob an electron. They aren't too fussy where they get one from and, usually, they have completed this task in microseconds.

Free Radical Rascals ...

These spare bits are called 'free radicals'. There is nothing sinister about the term 'radical'. It is derived from the Latin word for root, and its true meaning in English is 'essential' or 'fundamental'. When free radicals rob electrons, it is often from important components in the cells of our bodies. This causes physical damage to cells, often so comprehensively that they die. Scientists call this damage 'oxidative stress'. If you find that disturbing, consider this: every cell in your body – and you have trillions of them – sustains thousands of free radical hits every day!

Lest we be accused of implying that free radicals are nothing more than wanton nasties, let us make it clear that free radicals in our bodies are not all bad. In fact, they are essential to life itself. About three and half billion years ago, they responded to the intense solar radiation of the time to form the first complex organic molecules. But today, in the body, they are continually more active than is required, which is why the body needs also to produce antioxidants. These agents neutralise free radicals by donating the spare electron the free radicals are seeking, thus neutralising them, or by accepting the unpaired electron from the free radical.

This business of robbing single electrons raises a question. If free radicals rob electrons from other atoms, does that leave those burgled atoms with a lonely electron? Not always .... but, yes, it can. Turning the robbed atom into a free radical? You guessed it. A chain reaction! Things could run out of control pretty quickly, and that is why the body maintains its cellular army of antioxidants.

The discovery of free radicals and their activity in all living organisms has been a breaking story in medicine over the last 50 years or so. In that time, their place in science has evolved from a not very interesting fringe theory into a cornerstone of much current medical research. It is now believed they are responsible, at least in part, for over 100 diseases of the human body including AIDS and Alzheimer's. Moreover, the skin, eye, gastro-intestinal and immune systems are widely thought to benefit from the curbing of free radical activity. Allergic reactions and joint inflammation are also on the list. Chapter 5 discusses this in more detail, but let's take a quick look at the disease that kills and debilitates more humans than any other single condition, atherosclerosis.

Atherosclerosis – the Nightmare of the Congested Bypasses ...

This is caused by agglomerations of material, called plaques, developing on the inner walls of the arteries, restricting blood flow. Arteries form the high pressure pipe system of the body which carries freshly-oxygenated blood from the heart to all the organs. Atherosclerosis is thought to begin developing in Western people very early in life as faint fat deposits on the inner artery walls. Later, plaques develop, though not necessarily in those fatty spots. Of course, cholesterol has long been implicated in this disease but reducing cholesterol intake is not the key to its prevention, although it certainly can help. The little carriers that transport cholesterol around in the blood stream are called lipoproteins. You can have low density lipoproteins (LDLs) and high density lipoproteins (HDLs). LDLs are so called because they contain high levels of cholesterol and low levels of protein in contrast to HDLs which carry low levels of cholesterol and high levels of protein, which is far more preferable. Now, it has been established that LDLs can more easily shed some of their cholesterol at plaque sites, helping those to grow, if they have first been oxidised by free radicals. So we can see that free radical activity, while not the direct cause of heart disease, now stands convicted of setting off the chain of events that leads eventually to it.

Obviously, this is an over-simplified explanation. There is much literature and new thinking regarding the role of free radicals in the development of many of the most significant human diseases including cancer. The link between free radicals and cancer is still rather tenuous. The difficulty with cancer is that its roots lie in the most fundamental and least understood dimensions of our bodies, but it is becoming increasingly clear that even our DNA double helixes suffer irreparably from free radical attack. This is very difficult territory to investigate. In comparison it is far easier to observe how free radicals can be a factor in atherosclerosis and all of its dangerous consequences for the heart, the brain and other vital organs. A problem researchers have with free radicals is that most of them exist for only tiny fractions of a second – one researcher described their life cycle as "vanishingly brief" – so the study of their behaviour is exceedingly difficult.

The Avalanche of New Studies, New Information ...

Nevertheless, exciting progress is being made almost daily. We are starting to realise that free radical activity may be the cause of osteoarthritis, as it attacks tissues in our bone joints. Worse, it's equally likely that the inflammation thus caused kicks off further free radical formation. The unmasking of the free radical now even extends to the possibility that it may also be accelerating ageing. Researchers are not suggesting that if we crack this one, we will all live forever. The human life span is etched deeply in our genes, and interference with that dimension raises serious ethical questions. The recent debate on human cloning highlighted the widespread feeling that there are some places human technology should not dare to tread.

What is being postulated is a heightened quality of life for a greater proportion of one's time on earth by the reduction of the degenerative effects of ageing. There is growing support for the theory of ageing that says our bodies follow a genetically-controlled programme that gradually reduces oxidative defences, including the absorption of antioxidants from our diet. In other words, free radicals are progressively given freer reign to degenerate our bodies. Current thinking has it that if their activity can be restrained, the body will remain healthier, and in good shape, for longer.

Wouldn't we all like to be able to look forward to playing golf, walking the hills and swimming in the sea well into our eighties? This is one of the promises of repressing uncontrolled free radical activity in our bodies.

Which is what this book is all about.

The Naturally Occurring Antioxidants ...

As we have seen, free radicals are kept in check to a degree by antioxidants produced within our bodies. However this does not happen to a sufficient extent, and these endogenous antioxidants (i.e. antioxidants produced in our bodies) must be reinforced by outside help. Additional antioxidants enter our bodies via our food. With the prevalence of the advice that we should eat more fresh fruit and vegetables, it should be no surprise that these are by far the richest source of antioxidants.

All plants produce antioxidants for the very same reason as we humans do: plants need them for their natural defence systems, and they have them in abundance. Mostly, these botanical antioxidants come under the generic term 'flavonoids'. (The terms flavonoid and bioflavonoid are today commonly used interchangeably; for the sake of consistency, only the former is used in this book.) When they were first discovered earlier this century flavonoids were thought to be vitamins and given the name Vitamin P until around 1950 when researchers concluded they had no nutritional properties. We now know they are produced in plants because they have antioxidant properties and work to protect their host plants in a variety of different ways. They impart certain physical characteristics to their plants as well – colour being one. Vegetables which are red or purple are so because of a particular flavonoid. The redness of deciduous tree leaves in the autumn is caused by a flavonoid. Over 4,000 different flavonoids have so far been described and there may be many more to come as antioxidant research intensifies. Flavonoids are exciting because for us they are by far the most accessible natural antioxidants. To enjoy their benefit, all we have to do is take more careful note of all that advice to eat more fruit and vegetables!

Some plants have flavonoids and other naturally occurring antioxidants in greater concentrations than others, a fact not lost on the shamans, the witch doctors, the apothecaries, the herbalists – call them what you will – of just about every early civilisation that has ever been studied. The more we discover about the presence of antioxidants in nature, the more the treatments prescribed by the ancients for a wide range of ailments are at last finding scientific validation. If those ancients had acquired a similar facility for countering the ravages of infectious diseases, who knows how, and at what rate, human civilisation might have evolved?

The Growing Free Radical Menace ...

As we prepare for the arrival of the third millennium, however, we must deal with a continuing explosion in the ambient free radical population. Not only do our bodies generate free radicals, but we live in an environment that is absolutely bristling with them and we ingest them in ever increasing quantities as our lifestyles become increasingly divorced from the conditions enjoyed by earlier civilisations:

- We eat fatty foods which increase the levels of LDLs in our blood. We have already seen how dangerous LDLs can be when they are oxidised by free radicals.

- Our typical diet contains high levels of preservatives and peroxides which are implicated in increased free radical levels in our bodies. Further, processed foods lose a significant proportion of their antioxidant content during manufacturing.

- We are exposed to increasing levels of UV radiation due to thinning of the ozone layer; ultra-violet causes formation of free radicals in our skin layers. It is becoming increasingly likely that these UV-induced free radicals are at the root cause of melanoma.

- We are exposed to, as well as natural free radical sources, many free radical-forming influences such as radiation, microwaves, x-rays and magnetic fields. While these are not present in our usual environments to harmful levels, they can over a period of time tip the balance in favour of free radicals. Short-wave electromagnetic radiation, for example, can split water in the body to generate the hydroxyl radical, one of the most dangerous of them all. Radon, a natural radioactive gas, can reach possibly harmful levels in houses as it diffuses up from the ground. This too can cause free radical damage.

- In the room where you sitting now, it is likely that the coverings or coatings on the ceiling, the walls, the floor and the furniture are constantly emitting free radicals because of the degradation of the residues of the many chemicals that were used in their manufacture.

- Either directly or passively, we ingest cigarette smoke which is known to contain one of the densest free radical populations of any compound we might ever take into our systems. Most free radicals live for only a fraction of a second, but the semiquinone radical created by tobacco smoke can last several days.

- We breathe in motor vehicle emissions which, together with other forms of industrial pollution, are also a rich source.

- We subject ourselves to stress ... and we exercise. Yes, even excessive exercise bolsters the free radical assault on your body. For one thing, when you exercise you can use up to 20 times more oxygen than when you are not. Athletes and those on stringent exercise regimens, then, need to be especially aware of the heightened free radical activity in their bodies.

Free Radicals in our Lifestyles

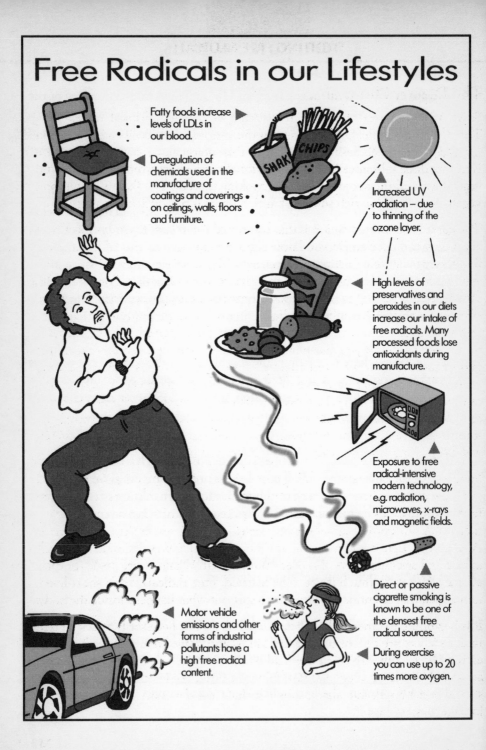

Fatty foods increase levels of LDLs in our blood.

Deregulation of chemicals used in the manufacture of coatings and coverings on ceilings, walls, floors and furniture.

Increased UV radiation – due to thinning of the ozone layer.

High levels of preservatives and peroxides in our diets increase our intake of free radicals. Many processed foods lose antioxidants during manufacture.

Exposure to free radical-intensive modern technology, e.g. radiation, microwaves, x-rays and magnetic fields.

Direct or passive cigarette smoking is known to be one of the densest free radical sources.

Motor vehicle emissions and other forms of industrial pollutants have a high free radical content.

During exercise you can use up to 20 times more oxygen.

The Dietary Shortfall ...

So we need to be extra careful in ensuring we take an antioxidant-rich diet. This is not so simple. Levels present in the various food species are covered in Chapter 4 and much has been written on this subject alone. Suffice to say there is tremendous substance in the conventional wisdom regarding fresh fruit and vegetables, and the avoidance of overcooking thereof. The fact that fruits and vegetables are such a rich source of antioxidants is not difficult to appreciate.

The current recommendation is that we should eat at least five servings of fruit and vegetables per day. Do you know many people who do that? Anyway, even five servings per day might not be enough. There is a growing realisation that even an ideal diet is not sufficient to prevent free radicals attacking our cells, causing the many degenerative conditions that cause disease and the general effects of ageing. Researchers are beginning to think the optimum intake for free radical neutralisation is closer to 12 servings per day. In the US, it is recommended that males take nine milligrams of Vitamin E per day to maintain good health. Vitamin E is an effective antioxidant, but researchers now say even sedentary males need five times that amount to prevent excessive free radical damage. Medical scientists are usually very conservative when it comes to making such recommendations. Perhaps they don't want to scare people by sounding too extreme or outrageous, but these dose recommendations might well keep rising as more is learned about free radicals.

Increasing medical, scientific and public recognition of all of the above has led to a new industry in antioxidant supplementation, and an intensifying search for the most efficient means of balancing the effects of antioxidants and free radicals in our bodies. Initially, work focused on vitamin antioxidants such as A, C and E. Beta-carotene, lipoic acid and mineral antioxidation helpers such as zinc and selenium have also been studied. Many claims were made for their efficacy. However, much is yet to be learned. Free radicals are so short-lived, remember, that scientists still struggle to sort out what happens inside the body.

It is beginning to emerge that all antioxidants do not necessarily attack all free radicals (there are dozens of different kinds) and indeed many of them may be extremely selective. To cover the field comprehensively, it is preferable to take an ideal balance of a range of antioxidants. For a guide on how that balance should be achieved, and what it should include, the manufacturers of Enzogenol looked to nature itself.

The Quest for a Better Natural Antioxidant ...

In the early 1990s, a talented multi-disciplined team at the University of Canterbury, representing biochemistry, biology, organic chemistry, chemical and process engineering, free radical research and natural product processing, recognised the need for a more effective antioxidant. They started a project to identify the most pure, rich and natural source of antioxidant and to develop an environmentally-clean process for its extraction. They were a great deal more successful in their search for a pure source of natural antioxidant than they had dared hope, for in the bark of *Pinus radiata*, they found a mother lode of highly active antioxidants.

Bark of trees of all kinds, but especially evergreen ones, has featured in herbal remedies since time immemorial. Captain Cook is credited with being New Zealand's first brewer for making a 'beer' from manuka as a tonic for his crew, a practice followed by Western seafarers for about 200 years before Cook's time. In the light of what we now know, all this makes perfect sense. Bark is a tree's armour in the sense that it protects the body of the tree from bacterial and insect attack. Apart from its sheer physical toughness, it performs this function by also acting as a transport system. If you make a cut in a pine tree, the bark quickly delivers resinous compounds to the wound, covering it up and providing a platform for the tree to heal itself, which it does in a remarkably short time. Bark is rich in flavonoid antioxidants. And research has established that pine bark is particularly so. There is more detail on this in Chapter 7, but radiata pine is a particular star in this regard. Unfortunately, it had until very recently proved difficult to extract the essential antioxidant-bearing material from pine bark without the use of toxic solvents.

Trees must survive the ravages of the environment for decades so it is natural that they have evolved a superior defence system compared with fruits and vegetables – mostly 'one season wonders'.

The Canterbury University team's intensive research into novel extraction processes culminated in the building of a pilot plant which used only pure water in its process and whose only waste product, apart from water which is recycled back into the process, is a beautiful garden mulch. The antioxidant components of the extract are concentrated using a new molecular selection process. This extraction method ensures that a number of significant groups of antioxidants, lost in conventional solvent-based processes, are harvested in – and this is of extreme importance – exactly the same ratios to each other as exist inside the bark itself. It is breakthrough technology and patents are pending in a number of countries.

Meanwhile the project team had located a sustainable plantation of fast-growing radiata pine, in which especially active antioxidant production can be expected. It grows in the complete absence of pesticides and chemical fertilisers in the pure soil, water and air of New Zealand's sub-alpine environment. Laboratory analysis confirmed this was a unique and superior source of certain critical antioxidant-bearing flavonoids and proanthocyanidins, even when compared with other pine barks. Bark peeled from the logs harvested in this specialist forest is transported immediately to the Enzogenol production facility and processed while it is still fresh. The felling of the trees from a sustainable forest enables the manufacturers of Enzogenol to harvest important live inner tissue, something those making bark products from standing trees are unable to access; only the outer bark can be taken if the tree is to continue growing. Extensive laboratory testing has shown that Enzogenol is not only beneficial but has also passed all safety tests.

The development of Enzogenol is a landmark in the fight against free radicals in the human body. Not only does it provide the most complete complex of proanthocyanidins, organic acids, flavonoids, glycosides, esters and carbohydrates yet incorporated in a safe diet supplement, but it is as natural a product as a concentrated capsule could ever be – and it is manufactured by a process which inflicts no harmful effects whatsoever on the environment, nor leaves harmful residues in the product.

Chapter 2

In The Beginning ...

By Dr Kelvin Duncan

Imagine what the world was like 3.8 billion years ago. It was a place we would not be able to survive in. There was little free oxygen in the air. The land was barren, and the sea was full of simple organisms that did not use oxygen but lived in a nitrogen-rich world. It was an anaerobic or "reducing" world.

Atoms such as iron did not rust because there was no oxygen to cause rusting. There were no green plants, and all autotrophic organisms – those that produce their own food as green plants do today – obtained their energy by a variety of chemical metabolic mechanisms that are now much rarer. Heterotrophic organisms – those that eat other organisms – were common as they are today. We are heterotrophic since we cannot make our own food, but must rely on the food produced by autotrophs. The Bible's statement that "All flesh is grass" is perfectly true today, but in these early times there was no grass.

These anaerobic conditions persisted for a very long time, for at least as long as life has subsequently existed on dry land. It was, no doubt, a pleasant and predictable world for those denizens, even though we modern humans could not survive in it longer than a few minutes if we were to be transported back to those days. It had endured for aeons and during that time slow evolutionary progress was made.

Then, all at once, a single event occurred which radically altered the whole earth and brought disaster to those organisms that had been living so happily in their cosy world. What was this disaster? It was the evolution of photosynthesis and the development of green plants.

Green plants are such a major feature of our life and environment that we can hardly imagine a world without them. Yet they are relatively recent arrivals on earth. When they first evolved, they were brilliantly successful. They had the trick of fixing carbon dioxide to make complex organic molecules, which are polymers consisting of carbon-carbon links, using the energy in sunlight. There is a vast amount of energy in sunlight, but it is hard to tap. This is the great adaptation made by green plants. They evolved mechanisms to harness the energy in sunlight to make organic matter. They thereby gained access to a vast amount of energy which they then used to produce an equally vast quantity of organic matter. To say the photosynthetic organisms flowered is misleading, because flowering plants came very much later, but they certainly did flourish, to the extent that they displaced most previous autotrophs.

Have you seen any of the older autotrophs around? They are still here, but in very special places.

The evolution of green plants, however, was a disaster of the greatest magnitude for most living things on earth. In the process of photosynthesis, green plants took carbon dioxide and water into their bodies, stripped off the hydrogen and oxygen atoms and released free oxygen and water. It was the rapid injection into the air of vast quantities of this new molecule that caused profound and, for most then-living organisms, disastrous changes to the environment. The atmosphere filled up with the destructive, plant-produced molecule that we call oxygen.

It is destructive because it oxidises chemicals so readily. It is so reactive that it is doubtful it occurs in a free form on any planet where there are no green plants to continually renew it. Earth's atmosphere was very quickly and totally replaced by the frenzied activities of green plants within the incredibly short period of about 2,000 years. No one knows why green plants photosynthesise so frenetically, but they do. They tend to produce far more food than they themselves need, which is good news for all us plant eaters!

But the rapid production of this destroying gas caused vast extinctions amongst the anaerobes that had previously inhabited the planet. Some survived and can still be found in the small pockets of anaerobic environment that persist on earth, such as in bogs and swamps, in rapidly decomposing flesh, and in fumaroles and the like. But the face of the earth was drastically changed, and most of the earlier inhabitants died.

Most of the anaerobic heterotrophs would have died, too, unless they did two things. They needed to evolve air breathing but, even more importantly, they had to become tolerant of oxidation – to defend themselves against the oxidative ravages of free oxygen. Oxygen is so necessary for life now that it is hard to comprehend this world where the newly developed oxygen was a dreadful threat to continued life. Yet it was. Needless to say, our antecedents, and those of the innumerable species with which we now share this planet, were successful in developing defences. They also evolved new and highly effective means of using this new molecule and these were so successful that most organisms now depend on oxygen for their continued existence.

In the absence of defences oxygen would rapidly oxidise and thereby destroy our tissues. So what were these defences that organisms evolved to protect themselves against oxygen? My view is that they are the polyphenol systems that all living organisms have. 'Polyphenol' means containing more than one phenol group. Cut an apple and it browns. Sunbathe and you brown. Both of these "browning wounds" are thought to be due to free radical damage: one due to oxygen and the other due to ionising radiation. The browning is the result of the formation of protective compounds from polyphenolic precursors.

This universal defence mechanism – the presence of polyphenols – has been thought to be for warding off invading micro-organisms, but I think they have a more fundamental role in protecting the body, and were originally evolved to defend against oxygen-derived free radicals.

Later in this book you will learn about free radicals, how they are formed and what they do, but for now let me emphasise that oxygen can be very destructive. Any faltering in your defence mechanisms, through disease, poor nutrition, stress, overwork, or any one of the hundreds of causes for the body to become run down, could result in horrendous damage from the self-same gas that supports your very existence, oxygen.

I do not want you to give up breathing, but there are positive things you can do to help your body to avoid damage. Order your life to remove the causes of stress and so prevent the damage that it can lead to. Eat healthy food, especially plenty of green leafy vegetables and fruit that contain so many antioxidants. Try to eat these in as raw a state as possible. Get plenty of sleep. And, if necessary, supplement your diet with natural antioxidants.

Why insist on natural antioxidants? If I am right in supposing that we are protected by a universal defence mechanism, you can supplement your own defence by taking antioxidants derived from other organisms at no risk to yourself health-wise. Pine bark is a good source of natural, healthy antioxidants. Indeed it is a rich lode as it is full of natural and health-giving flavonoids. Bark needs to be such a rich source because it has to last a long time, it is close to the villain in the piece, oxygen, and on its inner surface it has very active tissue. There is no doubt that the polyphenols in bark have other functions, but their role as antioxidants is the most important from our perspective.

Chapter 3

Tree Bark and Traditional Medicine

by Larry Stenswick

Trees have provisioned man abundantly down through the ages. They have been a source of wood for shelter, transport, weapons of war and instruments of cultivation, not to mention fuel for cooking and heating. And of course they provide food: apples, cherries, figs, peaches, pears, citrus, breadfruit, coconuts, mangoes and dates to name but a few of the most common. Then there is the huge variety of nuts and such edible oils as olive and palm. Trees provide cinnamon, cloves, pepper and nutmeg to spice our food. Several times a day we take beverages like coffee and cola that are made from trees. We chew the gums of trees. The fix for chocolate lovers comes from trees. We read papers and magazines, and package our materials in cardboard, all made from trees. Man has thatched roofs with leaves of palms, has made clothes with tapa cloths and has woven fabrics from all manner of bark and leaves.

Down the ages from the time of the very ancients, in every corner of the world, humans have been, and will probably continue to be, dependent on a cornucopia from trees.

For many, the strong tie between trees and medicine will come as a surprise. Trees, and especially the bark, provide a myriad of traditional remedies which not only hark back to antiquity but also span the world's cultures. Tree bark is the basis of two of the most important drugs in the history of man, aspirin and quinine. Today tree barks are yielding almost incredible breakthroughs in the war against cancer.

Voyages of The South Pacific

It was a weary and weak crew that Captain Cook led into Pickersgill Harbour, Dusky Sound, in May 1773. According to the records of this, his second, voyage to New Zealand, many were sick and ailing but soon they were to become strong and vigorous again. Fresh provisions would have helped, but Cook also made a spruce beer by boiling equal parts of rimu and manuka twigs in water. This tonic is what cured his crew of scurvy[1]. It is likely he learned how to make this brew from the local Maori who had been using native trees for a host of external and internal treatments. For centuries, Maori had used the bark of rimu and manuka, or ti tree, to excellent effect by making them into a decoction, a water extract achieved by boiling or simmering for a much longer time than one would infuse, say, tea. Rimu bark was also used to make a healing infusion for the treatment of running ulcers and as a poultice for burns and scalds[2].

The Maori arrived in New Zealand during the great migrations of Polynesians across the Pacific, and it is likely they brought these healing traditions with them. They quickly adapted to the pharmacy they found in the forests here and they made use of many barks including kahikatea, kohekohe, kowhai and pohutukawa.

They used kahikatea bark for treating bruises, and an infusion of it was given both internally and externally as a sedative. A decoction of bark relieved diarrhoea and dysentery. Kohekohe is a true mahogany and is often called New Zealand cedar. Its medicinal uses were well known. "The young bark is said to contain a bitter principal having tonic qualities similar to quinine..." said the noted artist James Goldie[1]. It was taken to allay coughs and it was one ingredient in the treatment of skin eruptions and kidney disorders. The inner bark of the pohutukawa was applied externally to stop bleeding and promote healing. After steeping in water, it was a valued remedy for diarrhoea and dysentery.

The westward migration of the Polynesians colonised nearly every island in a triangle from Hawaii in the north to New Zealand in the south-west and to Easter Island in the east. While not homogeneous, Polynesians share a common language base and have similar cultures. Some trees are common to many of the places they settled; it is likely those early voyagers dispersed these as they practised their incredible navigational skill and seagoing capability. One widely distributed tree is the *Casuarina equisetfolia*. In Tonga it is known as toa and an infusion of its bark is used to treat mouth infections and stomach aches. In Tahiti young stems of the aito, as it is known there, is used in the treatment of diabetes and nervous disorders. Also known as toa in the Cook Islands, the tree's inner bark is commonly given as an infusion to infants with thrush and mouth sores, and occasionally to people of all ages with urinary tract ailments.

Another tree widely used is one from the Myrtaceae family, *Syzygium malaccense*. In Samoa, a bark infusion known as seasea is taken for urinary tract infections, and it is used externally for treating inflammations in which case it goes by the name hehea. As ka'ika it is used to treat thrush in the Cook Islands, while in the Hawaiian Islands 'ohi'a'ai is the juice from grated bark used for sore throats, bronchitis and, occasionally, cuts.

In Samoa, nineteen different barks are uses for various treatments, while the best known Tongan decoction, vai kahi, is a blend of seven tree barks[3]. A complete compilation of medicines made from trees and plants in Polynesia for medicine would be a long list, and a high proportion of the items would be made from barks.

In common with other hunter-gatherer societies the Australian Aborigines used healing plants including tree bark in conjunction with complex rituals. Unfortunately, much of their oral tradition was lost with the deaths of elders and the dispersal of tribal groupings. Although they lacked a metal technology to boil water, we do know they produced decoctions of barks and other botanicals using hot stones. In Queensland the fever bark (*Alstonia* spp.), also called Australian quinine, was taken internally to treat fevers. Research in more recent times found that one compound found in fever bark, reserpine, markedly lowers blood pressure and is prescribed throughout the world[4].

Chinese Traditional Medicine

The use of barks in China predates Polynesian applications and is far more diverse. Here, we have the benefit of a *materia medica*. Published over 2500 years ago, the *Shen Nung Pen Tsao Ching* listed over 360 medicinal drugs made from plants. This seminal work was expanded in AD 657 during the Tang Dynasty to include about 730 drugs, and it was updated again in 1578. These products are still an integral part of the traditional Chinese medicine which has undergone a revival throughout Asia and is now embraced by many in the west. The focus is on maintenance of well-being, and tree barks make a major contribution.

Folkloric Japanese medicine, although widely applied, did not develop into a separate system because of the introduction and rapid acceptance of the Chinese methods in the fifth century. Products and information flowed from China to Japan until the 17th century when Japan cut itself off. After that, some Chinese plants continued to be imported to make drugs which were otherwise unobtainable but the Japanese also substituted domestic plants that had been shown to offer similar therapeutic benefits[5].

The shelves of any Chinese herbal outlet carry a variety of barks, each with its own characteristics and specific uses. Perhaps the best known of them is cinnamon, the dried bark of *Cinnamomum cassia* of the *Lauraceae* family. Cinnamon is used for fever control, diarrhoea and menstrual problems, and to soothe indigestion. It is mentioned in the very earliest of written records, and it was widely traded between Asia and Europe. More recent work confirms its potency as an antiseptic and in reducing the insulin requirements of diabetics. *Magnolia obovata* and *Magnolia officianalis* barks are prescribed as a skeletal muscle relaxant, analgesic and antihypertensive. *Phellodendron amurense* and *P. chinense* are commonly used to treat both diarrhoea and inflammation[6].

Recent research in China and, more especially, Japan has pinpointed many of the active constituents involved in these treatments, clarifying the biochemistry and pharmacology, and thus substantiating their healing effects. Yet today only a small fraction of the myriad of complex compounds in bark has been identified.

The Indians of Asia and North America

The Indians of the Indian sub-continent and those of the Americas have little in common, but both used the bark of trees to treat and heal.

Asian Indians have a rich tradition of using plants. Ayuvedic medicine has evolved over the past 5000 years. It was recorded in Sanskrit poetry in 1500 BC. The first Ayuvedic medical school was founded about 800 BC by Punarvasu Atreya. He authored the major work *Susrita Samhita* which describes 1500 plants and 350 valuable medicines.

Barks are an important component of Ayuvedic practice. One of the best known, the bark of the arjuna tree (*Terminalia arjuna*) has been used for at least 3000 years. As a tonic it has been highly valued in the treatment of heart failure and oedema – fluid accumulation in the ankles and legs because the heart is not pumping adequately. This traditional use has been confirmed and is in pharmacological use by many healers including Western-trained doctors. Just as remarkable is the dried bark of the varuna tree (*Crataeva nurvula*) which for centuries has provided relief from kidney and bladder stones. This remarkable bark is now being used in the West to prevent stone formation and related urinary tract infections[4].

In the Americas certain trees and barks were considered by the native Indians to hold supernatural medicinal powers. Picture yourself around a Cherokee fire as the tale is told of the origin of medicine:

> The plant had a special relationship with Mother Earth, as the story goes, to give life and oxygen for the animals and humans to breathe. In the presence of the Sun, they developed many varieties with different energies and shapes so that humans could recognise them. The humans did very well at deciding names based on shapes. The Plant Clan in council decided that it would be helpful to have different tastes and colors because humans were still young and had a lot to learn. This was a very long council, as the plants decided to have a presence for the humans to learn Medicine. After all the Great One intended for the humans to be keepers of Mother Earth. It was decided in the council of the Plant Clan for all plants to be helpers to the human spirits from that day forward[7].

The Cherokee use pine bark for many remedies. These people feel specially connected in spirit to the pine, and uses it in important ceremonies. They also use it for many remedies and often blend it with other herbs to "give them strength". To the Cherokee "the pines are all our brothers with special gifts of healing".

Other barks were also brewed; hawthorn (*Crataegus monogyna*) was made into a tea and given to sports competitors to increase their circulation. It is still used today to lower blood pressure and as an antispasmodic. Other tribes used pine, too, and one of the most recorded instances is the use of silver fir (*Abies amabilis*) by the North Wakashan and Southern Tsimshian tribes of British Columbia. They brewed the bark to make a tonic and found it an effective treatment for stomach ulcers. The neighbouring Bella Coola tribe took the bark tea for stomach ailments and used it to good effect against tuberculosis. The Nitinaht Indians of Vancouver Island used an infusion of red alder and hemlock bark for internal injuries[8,9].

Cramp bark (*Viburnum opulus*) was used by the Meskawi people to relieve cramps and pain throughout the body, while the Penobscot tribe used it to treat swollen glands and mumps. Prickly ash bark (*Zanthoxylum americanum*) was chewed by

Indians to relieve toothache and rheumatism, while the inner bark of the slippery elm (*Ulunus rubra*) was used for coughs and digestive disorders by the Mohicans. It is now believed compounds in the bark cause a reflex action which increases the production of mucus of the urinary tract and provides a soothing effect[4].

One widely used Native Indian medicine has found a use that continues today. Casa sagrada is derived from the bark of the buckthorn tree. Europeans were so impressed by the mildness and efficacy of this drug that they christened it 'sacred bark'. It remains the most widely used purgative in the world as no synthetic substitute has been found to replace it[10].

Chinchona Bark and the Treatment of Malaria

The Incas and Callaways of Brazil, and other native Indians of South America had for centuries used various tree barks of which the lapacho was especially valued because it provided a potent tonic and treatment for a wide range of conditions[4].

While the native Indians of South America did use various tree barks for the treatment of disease it was the introduction of cinchona bark by early Jesuit missionaries that would revolutionise the treatment of malaria on that continent. Cinchona grew wild in Colombia, Ecuador and Peru, and the bark was first used to treat fevers in about 1630. The name cinchona is said to be derived from the Countess of Chinchon, wife of a viceroy, who was cured in 1638. The remedy became known as Pulvo de la Condesa and quickly gained a reputation which spread back to Spain as soon as 1639. Rapidly distributed by the Jesuits, it first appeared in the *London Pharmacopoeia* in 1677, as Cortex Peruanus, commonly known as Jesuit powder[6].

Initially, the bark was obtained by felling wild trees but by the 19th century the Dutch in Java and the British in India were already cultivating the species. It has since been spread to Africa and Central America.

Used today chiefly in the treatment of malaria, it is now known as quinine, the most important compound in the bark. In the past 300 years this single bark derivative has benefited more people than any other drug used thus far to combat infectious diseases. While quinine can be synthesised in the laboratory it is not economical to do so and the world still relies on harvesting the bark. While mainly used to kill the malaria parasite, it is also taken as a non-specific remedy for fever and pain.

Aspirin from White Willow Bark

Therapeutic application of the bark of the white willow can be traced back to more than 2,000 years to when Hippocrates, the Greek physician known as the father of medicine, recommended chewing on willow bark to relieve pain and fever. Other cultures, from those of the North American Indian to the English of the Renaissance, shared this practice[11].

The active ingredient, salacin, was first isolated in 1828 and gained its current name, salicylic acid, in 1838. It was stabilised into acetylsalicylic acid by a young German chemist on 10 August,1897. He was seeking a pain-relieving medication for his father's debilitating rheumatism. Marketed by Bayer two years later as aspirin, it quickly became the world's most popular pain reliever. Although proven in the role, it was not until nearly 70 years later that British pharmacologist John Vane discovered how acetylsalicylic acid actually worked. It inhibits the body's production of certain chemical mediators, prostaglandins, that promote inflammation and thereby cause pain. Vane received the Nobel Prize for Medicine in 1982 for this research breakthrough[12].

More recently aspirin has re-emerged as an analgesic capable of saving life through its proven ability to help prevent heart attacks and strokes. Research is continuing into using aspirin in the prevention of other diseases including some cancers, diabetes, migraine headaches and Alzheimer's.

Trees Don't Get Headaches

In a parallel development, new understanding of the important role salicylates play in tree defence mechanisms is just emerging. University of Wisconsin researchers have found that some aspen trees produce higher levels of aspirin-like compounds that can fight off attacks of the voracious gypsy moth[13]. Botanists in several companies have reported on the complex role salicylic acid plays in defence of plants. In time this may result in increased protection from various diseases. Scientists are just beginning to understand the complexities of the processes of biosynthesis and metabolism that allow trees to improve their resistance to developmental, environmental and genetic factors. Scientists working in the equivalent human field are at a similar stage.

Tree Bark and the War against Cancer

Tree-sourced phytomedical compounds have moved into the mainstream of medicine, perhaps most spectacularly in respect of the treatment of cancer.

Taxol is Bristol Myers' trade name for paclitaxel, a compound found in the bark of the Pacific yew tree which grows mainly in the North-Western United States. In the late 1980s, Squibb and an innovative extraction company devised a method to extract this compound. After tests, the United States government's Food and Drug Administration granted Bristol market exclusivity and this bark derivative has gone on to become a phenomenal hit in the chemotherapy treatment of breast cancer, with world-wide sales of nearly 1 billion US dollars[14].

This success is part of a massive undertaking by ethnobotanists and biochemists to search out other sources of cancer-fighting compounds, and the bark of trees figures highly in the search. Common trees known to have anti-cancer compounds include horse chestnut (*Aesculus hipocastarnum*), betel nut (*Areca catechu*), bitter barked tree (*Brucea antidysenterica*) and its cousin ya dan zi (*B. javanica*), *Combretum caffrum*, chuan po shi (*Cudrania cochindhinensis*) , euptelea (*Euptelea plyandra*), fagara tree (*Fagara macrophylla*), American gelsemium (*Gelsemium sempervirens*), ginkgo tree (*Ginkgo biloba*), Eastern red cedar (*Juniperus virginiana*), *Mallotus japonicus*, *Maquira calophylla*, *Matemus* spp. which include the spindle tree, *Paramichelia baillonii*, *Psorospermum fefrigugum*, bitter bark (*Simaba multiflora*), twining tree (*Stizophyllum reparium*),yew (*Taxus mairei*) and *Vismia* spp[15].

The search is going on all around the world and the link between traditional medicine and modern medicine is nowhere better shown than in the work of ethnobotanist Paul Cox who spent years in Samoa studying the rain forests and the use of local medicinal plants by that country's faith healers. In the mid 1980s he found that patients with yellow fever, a viral disease, were being treated with a brew prepared by steeping the wood of a rain forest tree called *Homolanthus nutans* in water. The active compound in this concoction, prostratin, has proved effective against HIV. Another Samoan extract, from the bark of the *Alphitonia zizyphoides*, has been found to double the life of lymphocytes, key players in the body's immune system[5].

Henry Ciolino, a staff fellow at the National Cancer Institute in Frederick, Maryland, found that quercetin, a flavonoid found in pine bark, appears to block the action of aryl hydrocarbons, a class of potent carcinogens. These industrial toxins are found everywhere in daily life[16].

At the University of Illinois, Professor John Pezzuto has recently discovered that butylinic acid which is found in the barks of white birch, European plane tree and an African tree called ziziphus, can kill melanoma cells. A French research team has made very encouraging progress with the same compound in the treatment of HIV-1, the AIDS virus[16].

On 09 May 1998, Christchurch's "The Press" reported a potential breakthrough with a new drug which kills tumours by starving them of their blood supply. Accelerated human tests of this new compound, combrestatin, are now underway. It is a derivative of the African bush willow tree!

By coincidence the "New Zealand Herald" on 12 May 1998 related the efforts of an Auckland tree crop enthusiast to grow the Chinese *Camptotheca accumiata* tree, the bark of which has been used successfully in the United States to treat pancreatic cancer. The New York Academy of Sciences is quoted as saying these bark-derived products could be "... the ultimate anti-cancer drugs when fully developed."

Conclusion

Traditional medicine has incorporated and adapted tree barks throughout history to treat a wide range of diseases. Elements of traditional folk medicine have been adopted into the mainstream on many occasions in the past. Now we see this happening again.

We are just beginning to understand the immense complexity and richness of compounds found in tree barks. Over the next few years scientists will almost certainly unlock the secrets of how these wonder nutrients actually work. It will be a process of relearning what has been known for centuries: that tree barks can be extremely valuable in the treatment and prevention of the diseases that ravage man.

References

1. MacDonald, Christina (1993), *Medicines of the Maori*, William Collins, Auckland.

2. Stark, Dr. Raymond, (1979), *Maori Herbal Medicines*, Viking Sevenseas Ltd. Auckland.

3. Whistler, Dr. W. Arthur, (1991), *Polynesian Herbal Medicine*, National London Tropical Botanical Garden, Hawaii.

4. Chevellier, Andrew, (1996), *The Encyclopaedia of Medicinal Plants*, Dorking Kindersley.

5. Griggs, Barbara, (1993), *New Green Pharmacy* (2nd Edition),Vermillion, London.

6. Evans, Charles William, (1989), *Trease and Evans' Pharmocognosy* (13th Edition), Balliere Tindal, London.

7. Garrett, J.T. and Garrett, Michael, (1996), *Medicine of the Cherokee*, Bear and Company, Santa Fe.

8. Turner, Nancy J,Thompson, Laurence C. and Thompson, M.Terry et. al.(1983), *Ethnobotany of the Nitinaht Indians of Vancouver Island*, British Columbia Provincial Museum, Vancouver.

9. Compton, Brian Douglas, (1993) *Upper North Wakashan and Southern Tsimshian Ethnobotany: The Knowledge and Usage of Plants*, PhD Dissertation, University of British Columbia.

10. Wyatt, Jean (1994), "The Roots of North American Medicine." *Indian Life* Magazine, Vol. 15, Number 3.

11. Graeda, Joe and Ferguson, Tom (1993), *The Aspirin Handbook*, Garden Enterprises, Melbourne.

12. Bayer Corp, (1998), *Aspirin Turns 100: The Full Story*, http://www.bayerus.com.

13. Press Release (1998), *Arboreal Self Defense*, Univ. of Wisconsin.

14. Barrett, William (1998), "Delaying Tactics", *Forbes Magazine*, March 23.

15. *Bio Tech Resources* (1997) http://www.biotech,chem.indiana.

16. Laino, Charlene, *MSNBC Health News*, http://www.msnbc.com.

Chapter 4

Flavonoids: The Gift from Plants.

by Joshna Dayal

Flavonoids and phenolic acids are some of the most widely occurring groups of the powerful polyphenolic compounds introduced in Chapter 2. They occur naturally in almost all parts of plants including the roots, wood, bark, leaf, fruit and flowers.

Animals are not able to produce flavonoids endogenously and only a few are capable of accumulating them in their bodies. Most, including humans, must get their supply of flavonoids and phenolic acids from plants. We get our flavonoids from fruits, vegetables, grains, seeds, nuts, and beverages such as wine and tea.

Flavonoids are diverse both in their characteristics and chemical structures. Over four thousand of them have been identified and some researchers estimate that there could be up to twenty thousand different ones present in plants[1]. The tocopherol group of compounds, better known as Vitamin E, share the same basic structure as flavonoids. They are fat-soluble and, giving them antioxidant properties, monophenolic. While often raised in discussions on antioxidants, they are not however nearly as potent in this regard as the polyphenolic flavonoids. The general structure of flavonoids, which are generally based on a C_6-C_3-C_6, or diphenylpropane, skeleton, is shown below:

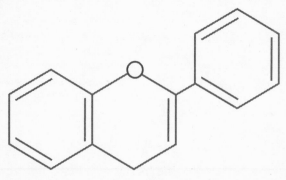

Figure 1. The generic structure of flavonoids

Technical Stuff

Flavonoids are widely occurring polyphenolic compounds, which have various biochemical activities. Polyphenolic compounds are those that have more than one phenol ring. All flavonoids are based on the basic C6-C3-C6 diphenylpropane skeleton.

Each intersection is actually a carbon atom (denoted by its chemical symbol "C"). Each carbon is able to form four bonds with carbon or other kinds of atoms, so the rings of the general flavonoid skeleton will actually look more like this:

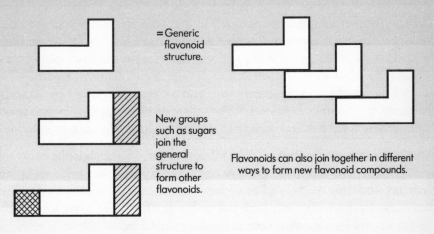

The flavonoids are divided into subgroups according to their oxidation level of the central pyran ring (C). The sub-groups of flavonoids include: flavonols, flavones, flavanones, catechins (flavanols), anthocyanins, proanthocyanidins, chalcones, isoflavonoids and aurones.

Flavonoids within these groups can also differ widely from each other. Other molecules such as sugars and hydroxyls are easily added (substituted) to the basic flavonoid structure in varying amounts and in varying positions.

For example if this block represents the generic flavonoid structure

= Generic flavonoid structure.

New groups such as sugars join the general structure to form other flavonoids.

Flavonoids can also join together in different ways to form new flavonoid compounds.

So, as you see the number of flavonoids that can exist is almost endless.

The flavonoids are separated into twelve main sub-groups by their structural class, and are further divided according to the arrangement and number of hydroxyl or any other groups present. The main groups of flavonoids are flavonols, flavanones, flavones, anthocyanidins and catechins. Some flavonoids exist as flavonoid glycosides, which means they have a carbohydrate, or plant sugar, attached. The glycoside is removed from the flavonoid in the gut during digestion. Flavonoids that do not have a glycoside molecule attached are called aglycones.

Simple flavonoids are able to join together to form other flavonoids. Take, for example, a very simple group of monomeric, or single unit, flavonoids called catechins. Catechins are found in many fruits and spices such as cinnamon and nutmeg, but in vegetables they are found only in rhubarb. There are several different types of catechins and they are able to bond together in a number of various ways to form different compounds that have very different characteristics. Two catechins joined together are called a dimer, and three catechins bonded together are called a trimer and so on up to oligomers and polymers. These new compounds are called proanthocyanidins, or condensed tannins. Catechins are the building blocks for proanthocyanidins and the number of the latter that can exist is almost endless.

Flavonoids are universally produced in plants for a number of reasons including protection against fungal parasites, herbivores, pathogens, oxidative cell injury and environmental stress[2]. Flavonoids also enable plants to make the bright colours that attract insects and promote pollination. So flavonoids are multi-functional, and their purpose may vary depending on the stress placed on its host plant and its stage of growth and development. Anthocyanidins which provide the vivid colours in many plants also act as anti-microbial agents within the plants, for example. In essence, flavonoids are a plant's defence system against environmental stresses and other factors that might inhibit its growth.

Another important group of polyphenolic compounds is the phenolic, or organic, acids. They are divided into two types, hydroxybenzoic acids and hydroxycinnamic acids, and are found in fruits and other plants. Their distribution varies with species, cultivar and stage of growth. Precursors of other flavonoids, they play a clear role in the nutritional value, colour, texture and taste of the fruit as well as its keeping qualities.

There are very good reasons humans should eat plants and plant products. Just as flavonoids and other phenolic compounds offer protection to plants, they can also protect us humans. It is well known that diets rich in fruit and vegetables provide protection against cardiovascular disease, certain forms of cancer and other diseases. As mentioned above, animals must get their flavonoids from plants because they are unable to produce their own. This could be another very good reason animals and plants exist so well together. By acting as antioxidants, flavonoids and phenolic acids protect us against the effects of free radicals and other mechanisms that can contribute to disease.

In Which Plants?

The concentration of flavonoids and related compounds in plant tissues varies considerably. One plant species can contain ten or more phenolics in differing concentrations. Generally, the leaves, flowers, fruits and other living tissues of plants contain glycosides while woody tissues contain aglycones. The seeds may contain phenolics in either form.

The skin, flesh and peel of fruit contain varying concentrations of flavonoids. The concentration changes with ripeness and storage. Catechin content of an unripe apple, for example, can be up to ten times higher than at maturity. Storage of fruit causes flavonoid levels to drop even further. Interestingly, plants grown under glass have lower flavonoid levels than those grown outside[3].

In general, flavonoid levels are lower in processed foods by around 50% than in fresh produce[4]. Flavonoids and phenolic acids are removed during handling, skinning and peeling. Although they are stable compounds with some resistance to heat, oxygen and moderate degrees of acidity, some are still lost during cooking[3,4].

It is quite difficult to list the flavonoids and the amounts typically present in the human diet. This differs according to the types of foods eaten and the variability of flavonoids in plants from region to region and country to country. Other varying factors are cultivar, growing conditions and degree of plant maturity. We may not be receiving a constant level of flavonoids from the food we eat, and certainly not the optimum level our bodies require. Table 1 shows the relative concentration of some common flavonoids and related compounds in plants[4,5].

Level of Flavonoids*in Fruit and Vegetables	
Low (< 10 mg/kg)	Cabbage, carrot, cauliflower, cucumber, mushroom, pea, peach, spinach.
Medium (Between 10 mg/kg and 50 mg/kg)	Apple, apricot, broad bean, grape, leek, lettuce, red pepper, strawberry, tomato.
High (> 50 mg/kg)	Broccoli, endive, French bean, kale, onion.
*quercetin, kaempferol, myricetin, luteolin and apigenin	

Table 1. Flavonoid content of some fruit and vegetables

Flavonoids are considered to be semi-essential nutrients and the average intake of flavonoids by humans is estimated at 23-170 mg/day[2]. Studies conducted in the Netherlands found that some of our main dietary sources of flavonoids are apples, onions, tea and red wine. There are no recommended levels for the flavonoid intake of humans at the moment and, as you can see from the table above, one has to eat a lot of fruit and vegetables to obtain reasonable levels of these important compounds. Another thing to consider is that not all fruit and vegetables contain either the same flavonoids (see table 2) or flavonoids at similar proportions to each other. For optimum health we not only need an acceptable level of flavonoids but, equally importantly, a good range of different flavonoids and organic acids. So, in terms of the fruit, vegetables and grains we need to eat every day, variety is just as essential as quantity.

Impact of Flavonoids on our Health

As we saw in Chapter 3, flavonoids from many plant sources have been used all around the world as medical treatments for many ailments and disorders. They possess outstanding properties and they should be considered as health-promoting and disease-preventing substances. It is likely the success of medicinal plants and their preparations relies not on single flavonoids but on the complex mixtures of the different compounds[9].

Source	Flavonoid Subgroup	Identified Compound
Apple	Flavonol Catechin (Flavanol) Proanthocyanidin	Quercetin (+)-Catechin, (-)-Epicatechin Procyanidins
Onion	Flavonol	Quercetin
Citrus Fruits	Flavanone Flavone Flavonol	Taxifolin, Naringin, Hesperidin Tangeretin Quercetin glycosides
Broccoli	Flavonol	Quercetin, Kaempferol
Celery	Flavone Flavanol	Apigenin Quercetin
Cherry	Anthocyanin Catechin (Flavanol) Proanthocyanidin	Cyanidin (-)-Epicatechin Procyanidin B1, B2, B5
Tomato	Flavanone Flavonol Phenolic acids	Naringin, Hesperidin Quercetin, Rutin, Quercetrin p-Coumaric acid
Spinach	Phenolic acids	Ferulic acid, Caffeic acid, p-Coumaric acid
Barley	Catechin (Flavanol) Proanthocyanidin Phenolic acids	(+)-Catechin Procyanidin B3 Ferulic acid, Vanillic acid, Protocatechuic acid
Strawberry	Proanthocyanidin	Procyanidins
Raspberry	Flavonol Anthocyanin Phenolic acid	Quercetrin Cyanidin p-Coumaric acid
Red Bell Pepper	Flavone	Luteolin

Table 2.   Sources of flavonoids[6,7,8]

Research into the effects of flavonoids on human health has really taken off over the past two decades. Flavonoids first came into the spotlight back in the 1930s when Szent-Györgyi and his colleagues extracted two flavonoids from citrus fruit. They investigated their effects and found they decreased capillary fragility and permeability in humans. Thus flavonoids were called 'Vitamin P' – f or permeability. This was probably the first study on the effect of flavonoids on human health but the work of Szent-Györgyi could not be repeated so the claim that flavonoids were vitamins could not be substantiated and the term Vitamin P was dropped around the 1950s.

Since then flavonoids have been reported in both *in vitro* and *in vivo* systems over a number of years to possess a huge array of biological effects, countering inflammatory, bacterial, viral, microbial, hormonal, carcinogenic, neoplastic and allergic disorders[10]. Flavonoids exert these antioxidant effects by neutralising all types of oxidising radicals[11] including the superoxide[12] and hydroxyl[13] radicals, and by chelation. A chelator is a compound which binds to metal ions in our bodies to prevent those ions being available for oxidation. Flavonoids are also able to act as powerful chain-breaking antioxidants due to the hydrogen-donating capacity of their phenolic groups.

Depending on their structure, flavonoids can be anti-allergenic. Quercetin has been found to inhibit histamine release. Histamine is what causes sneezing, watery eyes, itchy noses and other allergic reactions. Quercetin also inhibits the stimulated release of inflammatory 'mast cells' and other substances that contribute to the pathogenesis of diseases such as asthma, allergic conditions and others. Flavonoids are also known to be able to modify the activities of enzyme systems involved in a number of functions such as immunity, carcinogenesis, cellular transformation, tumour growth and metastasis. Certain flavonoids act against the enzymes that are critically involved in the life cycle of human immunodeficiency virus[14,15].

Cancer incidence is continuing to rise. In 1994, it caused over 25% of all deaths in Australia and New Zealand and while, we do hear of breakthroughs in the treatment of cancer, there has been little change in the mortality rates of cancer over the past 20 years. Some fruits and vegetables have been shown to decrease the risk of cancer. Flavonoids can act as blocking agents, inhibiting carcinogenesis. They do this in a number of ways, such as inhibiting the metabolic action of carcinogens by promoting enzymes that detoxify them, and by binding to carcinogens, preventing them from interacting with critical targets such as DNA and proteins. Flavonoids inhibit *in vivo* experimental carcinogenesis. In female rats, for example, a 50% reduction in the number of tumours was observed after feeding them a diet containing 5% quercetin. Flavonoids can also inhibit tumour promoters involved in carcinogenesis[15].

In this context, phenolic acids are important not only as the precursors of the other flavonoids found in plants but also because of their biological activity as antioxidants. Phenolic acids such as caffeic acid, gallic acid and others act as free radical acceptors and have been observed to inhibit mutagenesis and carcinogenesis[9].

Flavonoids and Coronary Heart Disease

Coronary heart disease is one of the biggest killers in the Western world today. In New Zealand and Australia, it accounts for approximately 24% of all deaths. Developments in cardiovascular disease research have shown that oxidative reactions and free radicals play an important role in myocardial injury and atherogenesis. Oxidation of low-density lipoproteins leads to their absorption by macrophages, a type of white blood cell which ingests foreign matter and thus plays a key role in the body's infection defence system. This macrophage absorption of oxidised lipoproteins promotes the formation of foam cells which in turn causes plaque to grow on arterial walls. Flavonoids reduce the oxidation of low-density lipoproteins and also prevent platelet aggregation by inhibiting the activity of the enzyme cyclooxygenase. Both processes are thought to lead to atherosclerosis and thrombotic tendencies.

The Zutphen Elderly Study[16], briefly referred to above, was an epidemiological study conducted in the Netherlands from 1985 to 1990. It investigated the relationship between dietary flavonoid intake and coronary heart disease. The flavonoid intake of over 800 men aged between 65 to 84 years was studied and determined to be 26 mg/day. The main sources of flavonoids were from tea (61%), onions (13%) and apples (10%). It was found that there was a significant inverse correlation between mortality due to coronary heart disease and flavonoid intake (see figure 2). In other words, fewer of those who ate larger amounts of flavonoids died of heart disease than those who consumed less. This result was still significant after adjustments were made for age, smoking, physical activity, coffee consumption and intake of Vitamins C and E.

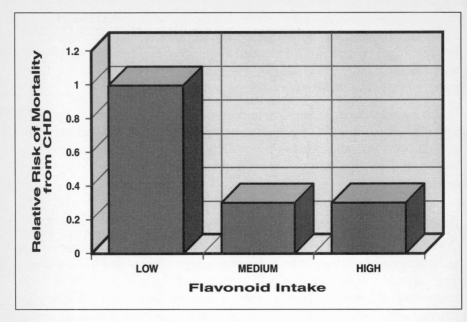

Figure 2. Relative risk of mortality from coronary heart disease and flavonoid intake, adjusted for age, diet, and other risk factors[16].

This is further supported by the Seven Countries Study[5] in which the main objective was to determine whether flavonoid intake explained differences in mortality rates from chronic diseases across populations. It concluded average flavonoid intake might contribute to differences in mortality from coronary heart disease.

Flavonoids and Strokes

A recently published study investigated the intake of antioxidants, including flavonoids, on the incidence of stroke. Dietary flavonoids were again inversely associated with stroke incidence after adjustment for age, systolic blood pressure, serum cholesterol, smoking, energy intake and consumption of fish and alcohol. This indicated the more flavonoids you consume, the lower the risk of stroke. The study showed intake of Vitamin C and Vitamin E was not associated with stroke risk.

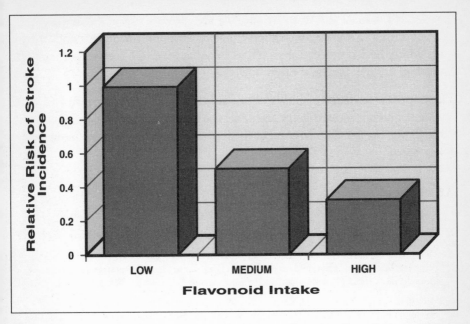

Figure 3. Relative risk of stroke incidence and flavonoid intake adjusted for confounding factors[17].

Flavonoid Supplementation Required

Health trends and health care have changed, and will continue to do so. No longer are infectious diseases such as tuberculosis, and bronchitis major threats to our lives. We are living longer, but we are now falling ill to age-related diseases such as cancer, heart disease, and neuro-degenerative diseases like Alzheimer's.

We do not have cures for all 'modern diseases', and treatment comes after the disease has arrived. Unfortunately, there is very little emphasis on the prevention of disease. Vegetables, fruits and cereals are not only our major sources of vitamins, minerals and carotenoids but also of flavonoids and other related phenolic compounds that play an important role in human health. Flavonoids occur in many of the foods we should be eating but in today's hectic world it is not always easy to obtain desirable levels of antioxidants and flavonoids through the diet. It is harder still to make sure we are eating a varied selection of fruit and vegetables so we receive a good range of different flavonoids and organic acids. Many health professionals tell us to eat at least five servings of fruit and vegetables per day but how often does this happen?

The importance of flavonoids to human health is becoming more and more apparent, and it is more than probable we are not consuming enough flavonoids through our regular diets to combat the free radical activity to which our bodies are exposed.

References

1. Colgan, M (1994)*The New Nutrition. Medicine for the Millennium*, C I Publications, San Diego.

2. Cook, N C, Samman, S. (1996) "Flavonoids - Chemistry, metabolism, Cardioprotective Effects and Dietary Sources." *J. Nutr. Biochem.*, Vol 7.

3. Peirpoint, W S. (1986) "Flavonoids in the Human Diet." From *Plant Flavonoids in Biology and Medicine: Biochemical, Pharmacological and Structure-Activity Relationships*, Alan R Liss.

4. Hertog, M G L, Hollman P C H, Katan M B. (1992) "Content of Potentially Anticarcinogenic Flavonoids of 28 Vegetables and 9 Fruits Commonly Consumed in The Netherlands." *J Agric Food Chem*, Vol 40.

5. Hertog, M G L, Kromhout, D, Aravanis, C, Blackburn, H, Buzina, R, et al,. (1995) "Flavonoid Intake and Long-term Risk of Coronary Heart Disease and Cancer in the Seven Countries Study." *Arch Intern Med*, Vol 155.

6. Kuhnau, J. (1976) "The Flavonoids. A Class of Semi-Essential Food Components: Their Role in Human Nutrition." *Wld Rev. Nutr Diet.*, Vol 24.

7. Rice-Evans, C. A., Miller, N. J., Paganda, G. (1996) "Structure-Antioxidant Activity Relationships of Flavonoids and Phenolic Acids." *Free Radical Biology & Medicine*, Vol 20, No 7.

8. Herrmann, K (1976) "Flavonols and Flavones in Food Plants: A Review". *J. Fd. Technol.* Vol 11

9. Pietta, P. (1998) *Flavonoids in Medicinal Plants. From Flavonoids in Health and Disease*, edited by C A Rice-Evans and L Packer, Marcel Dekker, New York.

10. Middleton, E. (1996) "Biological Properties of Plant Flavonoids: An Overview." International *Journal of Pharmacognosy*, Vol 34, No 5.

11. Bors, W, Heller, W, Michel, C. (1998) "The Chemistry of Flavonoids." From *Flavonoids in Health and Disease*, Edited by C A Rice-Evans and L Packer, Marcel Dekker, New York.

12. Robak, J, Gryglewski, R J. (1988) "Flavonoids are Scavengers of Superoxide Anions." *Biochemical Pharmacology*, Vol 37, No 5.

13. Husain, S R, Cillard, J, Cillard, P (1987) "Hydroxyl Radical Scavenging Activity of Flavonoids." *Phytochemistry*, Vol 26, No 9.

14. Kandaswami, C, Middleton, E. (1994) "Free Radical Scavenging and Antioxidant Activity of Plant Flavonoids." From Free *Radicals in Diagnostic Medicine*, Edited by D Armstrong, Plenum Press New York.

15. Middleton, E, Kandaswami, C. (1993) "The Impact of Plant Flavonoids on Mammalian Biology: Implications for Immunity, Inflammation and Cancer." From The *Flavonoids: Advances in Research since 1986*. Edited by J B Harborne.

16. Hertog, M G L, Feskens E J M, Hollman P C H, Katan M B, Kromhout, D. (1993) "Dietary Antioxidant Flavonoids and Risk of Coronary Heart Disease: the Zutphen Elderly Study." *Lancet*, Vol 342.

17. Keli, S O, Hertog M G L, Feskens E J M, Kromhout D. (1996) "Dietary Flavonoids, Antioxidant Vitamins and Incidence of Stroke." *Arch. Intern. Med*, Vol 156.

Chapter 5

Free Radicals – More than Revolutionary

by Dr Steven Gieseg

Over the past few years, free radicals have been implicated in all sorts of diseases. Every health supplement seems to include some protection against them – but what are they and, more importantly, what do they do?

We first need to go back to high school chemistry to understand what a free radical is. All atoms contain a nucleus which is made up of protons and neutrons, and electrons move around this nucleus. The chemical bonds which hold different atoms together to make molecules contain pairs of electrons. The hydrogen molecule (H_2) for example, has two electrons in each of the bonds

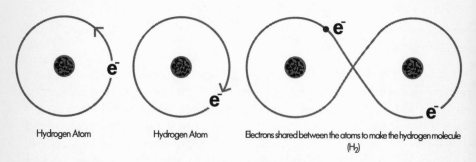

| Hydrogen Atom | Hydrogen Atom | Electrons shared between the atoms to make the hydrogen molecule (H_2) |

Figure 1: The hydrogen molecule, H_2. Electrons are shared between the atoms. This is often written as H:H to show the shared electrons making the bond.

holding the hydrogens together. In the water molecule (H_2O) there are two electrons in the bonds holding the hydrogens to the oxygen. The two electrons act to stabilise the bond between the atoms.

However some molecules, especially those containing oxygen, can easily gain only one of these bonding electrons which means that it then has an unpaired electron. The fact that this electron is not paired with any other electron makes it very reactive. This is essentially what a free radical is: a molecule containing unpaired electrons. This molecule will steal electrons from other molecules in order to pair its lone electron. In doing this it changes the structure of the other molecule and could even turn that molecule into another free radical.

Free radicals are produced within cells continuously as by-products of normal metabolism breaking down food molecules to release cellular energy. White blood cells also produce free radicals when they work to protect the body by killing and breaking down bacteria and other nasties that pose a threat to our well-being. There are several different types of free radicals which can form within our bodies. They can react with many of our bodies' chemicals and may cause damage to important metabolic processes. For example, damage to DNA could result in genetic mutations or the switching on of growth genes causing cells to become cancerous.

The Hydroxyl Radical

The most reactive radical molecule known is the hydroxyl radical. It can be made by X-rays or gamma rays from radioactive isotopes hitting water molecules. The rays cause one of the bonds holding the hydrogen to a oxygen to split in half. One electron of the bonding pair goes to the oxygen and the other to the hydrogen as shown in Figure 2.

The resulting hydroxyl radical, written HO to show the lone electron, is so reactive that it takes only a billionth of a second to react with a neighbouring molecule and it can cause a lot of biological damage. What usually happens is it regains its lost electron by taking a hydrogen atom from another molecule. If that molecule happens to be a piece of DNA the effect could be a genetic mutation leading to the switching on of a cancer gene. So in a sense, nuclear radiation such as gamma rays do not actually cause mutations; it is the free radicals generated from the water in the body which cause the damage.

45

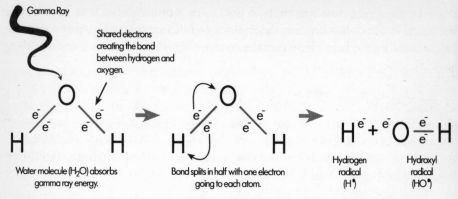

Gamma Ray

Shared electrons creating the bond between hydrogen and oxygen.

Water molecule (H_2O) absorbs gamma ray energy.

Bond splits in half with one electron going to each atom.

Hydrogen radical (H˙)

Hydroxyl radical (HO˙)

Figure 2: The effect of gamma rays on water molecules. One of the energised water molecule's hydrogen-oxygen bonds splits in half, with one electron going to each atom. This produces one hydrogen radical and one hydroxyl radical.

Superoxide: the Good, the Bad, the ...

Thankfully, exposure to gamma rays is not an everyday event for most of us. That makes superoxide the most commonly encountered free radical in biology. Superoxide is an oxygen molecule with an extra unpaired electron and is usually written as O_2^- . Superoxide is formed in the body either deliberately by white

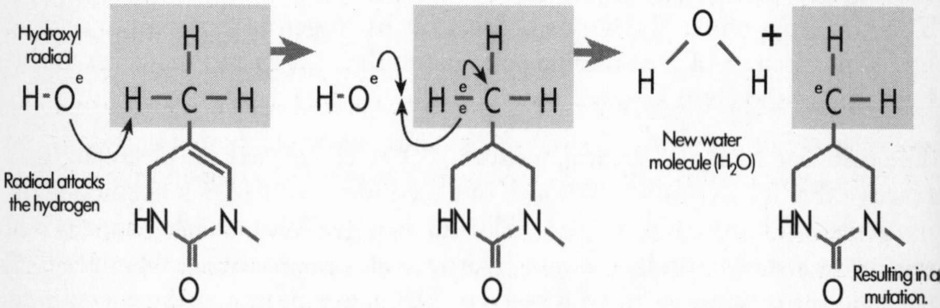

Hydroxyl radical

H-O˙

Radical attacks the hydrogen

New water molecule (H_2O)

Resulting in a mutation.

Figure 3: The hydroxyl radical attacking the thymine group in DNA. A hydrogen-carbon bond is split and a new bond forms between the hydroxyl radical's oxygen and the hydrogen. Thus, one hydrogen atom is stolen from the DNA by the hydroxyl radical and the DNA is left with a carbon radical, causing a mutation.

blood cells killing invading bacteria and viruses or accidentally as the leakage of energy when cells burn food molecules. In both situations it appears that the superoxide formed can cause changes to our bodies biological molecules leading to various forms of damage.

Superoxide from White Blood Cells

Major sources of superoxide are specialised white blood cells called macrophages and neutrophils. An enzyme present on the surface of these blood cells, NADPH oxidase, is switched on when the cells encounter invading foreign molecules, such as a bacterium. NADPH oxidase adds an electron to the oxygen molecules around it creating even more superoxide.

Superoxide is not actually that reactive and it usually reacts with itself to form a compound called hydrogen peroxide. Hydrogen peroxide is commonly used as hair bleach. It has no unpaired electrons so it is not a free radical but is called a 'reactive oxygen species', even though it is not, on its own, all that reactive. The problem with hydrogen peroxide is that it can very easily make more damaging hydroxyl radicals whenever an electron is supplied to it, making it a potential time bomb.

In addition to switching on the NADPH oxidase superoxide-producing enzyme, the neutrophil-type white blood cells also produce the enzyme myeloperoxidase. This enzyme is an amazing green colour in the test tube and most people are familiar with it as the green phlegm on their handkerchiefs during a bad head cold. Myeloperoxidase takes the hydrogen peroxide and the salt in your blood and converts it to hypochlorite, in other words chlorine bleach. Chlorine bleach is a potent and lethal killer of bacteria and, unfortunately, anything else it encounters including healthy cells. When unleashed on a cell it destroys the enzymes and structural proteins by adding chlorine atoms to them. The destruction of these enzymes causes the cell's metabolism to grind to a halt and the cell dies.

Hypochlorite is the heavy artillery of the reactive oxygen species so it's not surprising that other cells and body tissues often sustain damage when bacteria are killed by these white blood cells. Hypochlorite production, at the wrong time, in the wrong place or in excess has been implicated in a number of disease including those of the lung, and possibly, the heart. Researchers using specific chemicals which stain myeloperoxidase so it can be seen under the microscope have seen this enzyme in the fatty growths in the artery walls of patients with heart disease.

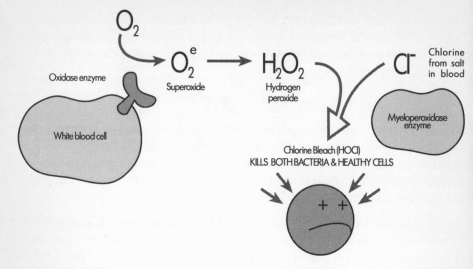

Figure 4: How white blood cells produce hypochlorite, more familiar to us as chlorine bleach, to fight invading organisms: the enzyme NADPH oxidase adds an electron to oxygen, converting it to hydrogen peroxide. With the help of another enzyme also produced by the white blood cells, myeloperoxidase, the hydrogen peroxide is converted into hypochlorite.

Superoxide as Energy Leakage

We like to think our body's machinery is perfect, but it is not. Five percent of the oxygen we breathe forms the free radical superoxide. The second major way we produce superoxide radicals is as leakage of energy during the burning of food molecules by our cells. The final stage of releasing energy from the foods we eat involves a series of reactions where electrons are passed from one molecule to the next, forming a type of electric current. One time out of twenty, one of the electron carriers, Coenzyme Q, passes the electron to an oxygen instead of the next electron carrier, producing superoxide.

This presents the body with a considerable problem. The large amount of superoxide produced will react with a nitrogen-containing messenger molecule called nitric oxide. Nitric oxide is the vital signal molecule which controls our blood pressure. The loss of nitric oxide through the reaction with superoxide is potentially lethal. As well, the resulting new molecule is another reactive oxygen species which can stick nitrogen groups to proteins and enzymes causing them to deactivate. Nitric oxide can also break down to the hydroxyl radical, resulting in even more damage.

The body prevents this from occurring by speeding up the reaction discussed earlier whereby superoxide reacts with itself to give hydrogen peroxide. It does this with a special enzyme called superoxide dismutase. This enzyme is found in all body cells and acts to dispose of the superoxide generated during energy production. However the product of this reaction is hydrogen peroxide which, as mentioned earlier, can cause further oxidative damage by acquiring an extra electron thus forming the more reactive and more harmful hydroxyl radical. Hydrogen peroxide can source this electron from the copper and iron in our bodies. The reaction is shown below and is known as the Fenton reaction after the man who first described it in 1893.

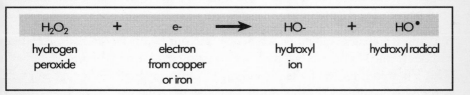

$$H_2O_2 \quad + \quad e^- \quad \longrightarrow \quad HO^- \quad + \quad HO^\bullet$$

| hydrogen peroxide | electron from copper or iron | hydroxyl ion | hydroxyl radical |

The body prevents the Fenton reaction in two ways. Firstly, it binds up all the copper and iron very tightly in special protein carriers, such as albumin, so they cannot react. Secondly, the hydrogen peroxide is broken down to water and oxygen by the enzyme catalase.

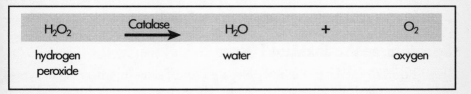

$$H_2O_2 \quad \xrightarrow{\text{Catalase}} \quad H_2O \quad + \quad O_2$$

| hydrogen peroxide | water | oxygen |

In this way the superoxide leaked from the energy-producing reactions within the cell is converted back into normal oxygen. The superoxide dismutase and catalase enzymes thus act together as antioxidant enzymes, breaking down the reactive superoxide and hydrogen peroxide to prevent free radical damage.

Antioxidants, our Protection against Disease

As you can see, the body creates free radicals and oxygen reactive species relentlessly and continuously. Antioxidants are compounds that provide the body with protection against their harmful effects. At low concentrations antioxidants are able to react with free radicals, forming harmless unreactive molecules and so protecting other biological molecules from damage. Humans can produce some antioxidants within the body, including specialised enzymes like the catalase and superoxide dismutase already discussed. To protect sites in the body the enzymatic systems cannot reach, antioxidants such as Vitamins C and E and flavonoids are obtained from dietary sources. These are rapidly turned over in the body and need to be constantly replenished. Antioxidants work in a number of ways to protect the body: decreasing the quantity of free radicals or reactive oxygen species produced, neutralising free radicals, binding metals to stop them from reacting and making more damaging free radicals, thus preventing degeneration

Vitamin E is an antioxidant which dissolves in our body's fats and oils. Any free radicals formed in the fats will react with Vitamin E to form a Vitamin E radical. This Vitamin E radical lacks the energy to cause any further damage but will react with Vitamin C in the blood, thus regenerating itself. The breakdown product of Vitamin C is removed by the kidneys. In this way the free radicals formed in fats are removed from the body by transfer to Vitamin E, then to Vitamin C and out through the kidneys as urine. Vitamin C also reacts with any water-soluble free radicals formed in the blood.

Certain flavonoids may interact with these antioxidants in a similar way to provide additional protection against free radical damage.

Selenium, an Antioxidant Helper

In addition to catalase, the body has a group of selenium-bearing enzymes collectively called glutathione peroxidase. These enzymes break down hydrogen peroxide and peroxides which form on the fats and oils within the body. It is called glutathione peroxidase because it transfers the energy of the free radical to a very small sulphur-containing protein called glutathione. The selenium inside the enzyme acts as the reactive centre, carrying the reactive electron from the peroxide to the glutathione. The glutathione is the antioxidant in this reaction, not the selenium. Certainly, selenium is an important trace element in our diet, being required for the synthesis of the glutathione enzyme. By itself, however, selenium is actually a potent oxidant which can generate free radicals. Only when it is built into the enzyme is its electron-carrying power used to prevent free radical reactions. Though it will take a lot of selenium to kill a person, only ten times the required daily intake will start to make the average person sick – by the very process they are taking selenium to prevent.

Free radicals: the friction wearing out the metabolic machine

For at least the first twenty or so years of our lives our bodies appear well protected from free radical damage. The levels of both antioxidant molecules and antioxidant enzymes are high enough to absorb most of the free radical fluxes occurring in the body during this time. As we get older the effectiveness of these protective systems slowly decreases. It seems not all the free radicals produced are neutralised and so there is a slow build-up of damaged molecules. The damage includes the antioxidant defence systems and so as we age there is a slow decrease in the amount of active superoxide dismutase, catalase and glutathione peroxidase operating in our bodies. Just as friction wears out a machine, free radicals wear out the body. The severe complications of life-long exposure to free radicals appear as diseases we associate with ageing:

Coronary heart disease

Coronary heart disease (atherosclerosis) appears to be caused by damage to the cholesterol-bearing particles in the blood. The damaged particle is taken up by white blood cells called macrophages which collect in the artery wall, forming plaques. The cholesterol-filled cells attract other cells causing a growth on the inside of the artery which slows or blocks the flow of blood to the heart. If the growth breaks open the blood will clot, blocking the flow of blood to the heart muscle and resulting in a heart attack.

Stroke

The same applies as for heart disease but in this case it is the arteries supplying blood to the brain that are affected.

Cancer

Free radicals react with cells' DNA causing mutations. If the free radical damage is not repaired the DNA sequence will change, causing mutations. This may result in the switching on of cancer-causing growth genes and the switching off of cancer-stopping genes within a cell. Usually a cell requires two or more genes to be altered before it becomes cancerous. The majority of cancers and other mutations are caused in this way.

Rheumatoid Arthritis and Chronic Inflammation

Inflamed joints have large numbers of active white blood cells present. These macrophages and neutrophils release damaging molecules such as hydrogen peroxide and superoxide. If the joint bleeds the iron level can be increased and hydroxyl radicals are produced, causing even more damage as well as pain and swelling.

Cataracts

The formation of cataracts involves the oxidation of the lens proteins. UV light and iron generate the free radicals which cause sugar molecules and other compounds to react with the lens proteins, forming coloured compounds that block the passage of light through the lens.

Alzheimer's

Damaged proteins build up in specific areas of the brain and the various neurons begin to die. A free radical mechanism may be at work.

Free Radical Research

The research into free radicals and their effect on cells is very complicated. Because they are very reactive, and therefore very short-lived, researchers cannot measure these radicals directly and must look for the damage they cause. Unfortunately, free radical reactions are messy. The hydroxyl radical can form more than a hundred different products when it reacts with a protein. With fats it is even more complex. Many of the products of free radical damage to fats are unstable and break down into even more complex compounds. The measurement of one of these compounds in the blood does not always mean the body is being permanently damaged; it could be that the body is dealing with the damage successfully by removing it. To make matters even more complex, diseases such as those of the heart develop over many years, a rate impractical to model in the test tube. Understanding these free radical processes within the complex machinery of the body is a difficult task.

The questions for medical science are whether increased antioxidant protection can slow this process and, if so, which antioxidant is the best? Some antioxidants in excess, for example Vitamin C, can themselves become oxidants, which is probably why the body tightly controls the concentrations of many of its antioxidants. Blood Vitamin E levels are so tightly controlled that, to double their Vitamin E level, average people need to increase their Vitamin E intake tenfold. In other words 90% of the expensive vitamin is literally going down the drain.

Many researchers and medical practitioners believe that increased dietary intake of antioxidants, by the consumption of fresh fruit and vegetables or dietary supplements such as flavonoids, Vitamin C and Vitamin E, can slow the processes of free radical damage and associated ageing diseases. Proving this, however, is a very slow and difficult process as these diseases take a long time to develop and we humans are all different, both in our lifestyles and genetics. Much of the research that has been carried out on dietary antioxidants has been focused on Vitamin E merely because of its early discovery. Evidence is coming in only now from the first of these studies. Trials are indicating that Vitamin E and flavonoids may have a protective effect against heart disease. Researchers claim that dietary changes designed to decrease the level of free radical reactions can reasonably be expected to increase the span of healthy productive life by at least five years.

The whole spectrum of antioxidants produced both in the body and those obtained from the food we eat interact with each other, providing a complex regulatory metabolic pathway. Plant flavonoids have exhibited remarkable properties and they should be considered natural dietary disease-preventing, health-promoting, substances. Several epidemiological studies have shown that increased consumption of fruit, vegetables and flavonoids reduces the incidence of coronary heart disease, cancer and stroke. Although the exact way in which plant flavonoids interact within the body, with each other or with other antioxidants is not yet fully understood it is likely play an important role in maintaining our health by lowering the degree of free radical damage to our bodies. Research into flavonoids and health continues to grow and the next decade will provide many of the answers we have been waiting for.

Further reading

Beckman, J. and Koppenol, W. H., (1996) "Nitric Oxide, Superoxide, and Peroxynitrite :the Good, the Bad, and the Ugly", *The American Journal of Physiology*, 271, C1424-C1437.

Cheeseman, K. H. and Slatter, T. F., (1993) "An Introduction to Free Radical Biochemistry", *British Medical Bulletin*, 49, 481-493.

Dean, R. T., Gebicki, J. M., Gieseg, S. P., Grant, A. J., and Simpson, J. A., (1992) "Hypothesis: a Damaging Role in Aging for Reactive Protein Oxidation Products?", *Mutation Research*, 275, 387-393.

Dean, R. T., Gieseg, S. P., and Davies, M. J., (1993) "Reactive Species and their Accumulation on Radical damaged Proteins", *Trends in Biological Science*, 18, 437-441.

Esterbauer, H., Puhl, H., Waeg, G., Krebs, A., and Dieber-Rotheneder, M., (1992) "The Role of Vitamin E in Lipoprotein Oxidation", in *Vitamin E in Health and Disease*, Edit L. Packer and J. Fuchs, Published by Marcel Dekker, Inc., 650-671.

Halliwell, B. and Gutteridge, J. M. C., (1989) "Free Radicals in Biology and Medicine", 2nd Edition, Clarendon Press, Oxford.

Kettle, A. J. and Winterbourn, C. C., (1997) "Myeloperoxidase: a Key Regulator of Neutrophil Oxidan Production", *Redox Report*, 3, 3-15.

Koppenol, W. H., (1993) "The Centennial of the Fenton Reaction", *Free Rad. Biol. Med.*, 15, 645-651.

Steinberg, D., Parthasarathy, S., Carew, T. E., Khoo, J. C., and Witztum, J. L., (1989) "Beyond Cholesterol Modifications of Low-density Lipoprotein that Increase its Atherogenicity", *The New England Journal of Medicine*, 320, 915-924.

Chapter 6

From *Pinus radiata* to Enzogenol
by Ian Gilmour

Scientists and engineers are being challenged to invent and design clean technologies to replace established ones which tend to be, in the main, polluting. Very few industrial processes can be considered to be clean in their execution. Clean means green, where there are no waste streams, only useful by-products which benefit humanity and the environment.

The growth of a tree is the ultimate in clean technology. A tree can be considered to be a biological factory. The seed represents the capital plant and investment. The raw materials are sunlight, atmospheric carbon dioxide, water from both atmosphere and soil, and mineral nutrients from the soil. The main product is the tree itself, a storehouse of components and compounds, and the major by-product is oxygen which is released to the atmosphere. Definitely a good role model to emulate!

In centuries past trees were prized for entirely different reasons. A nation's military might was gauged by the size of its naval fleet. Trees were a treasury of timber and chemicals for ships and naval supplies, so forests were considered to be a country's most valuable resource. Tall straight conifers were highly valued for masts. Britain and Spain searched the world for colonies with tall, straight and mature pines. They were interested in forming new colonies in South America, Australia and Norfolk Island mainly because of their magnificent virgin forests of mature conifers. Oaks were used for hulls and superstructures. Governments had to order ahead and allow 100 years for oaks to mature for ship building.

Trees and woody plants provided most other materials for maintaining a naval fleet as well. Jute, hemp, flax and cotton were used for sails and rigging. Distilled wood products such as creosote and tar, wood alcohol and charcoal provided timber preservatives, solvents and fuels. The technology for producing these

55

was well-known and quite well-documented up until the1930s but practical engineering know-how and literature on it faded as iron and steel gradually displaced wood as a construction material for ships.

At the turn of this century, oil replaced wood as a source of energy and chemicals. A nation's military strength and wealth then became dependent on ownership of oil and iron reserves. Interest shifted from forest-rich colonies to oil-rich ones. Trees lost their dominance and worth as assets.

Today, forests are valued for their role in stabilising the ecology and climate of the globe by helping to maintain its carbon balance. Trees use and store carbon so they serve as sponges, soaking up surplus carbon dioxide emissions from human creations such as thermal power stations and motor vehicles. Carbon dioxide is one of the main greenhouse gases, insulating the earth and causing global warming. Of course, trees still provide timber for buildings, raw material for paper, fuel and a source of resins. As Chapter 3 explained in fascinating detail, the bark of trees continues to yield a wealth of natural medicines and drugs.

But there is no longer whole tree utilisation by a naval stores industry. Only the pulp and paper industry comes close to doing this but its focus is very much on paper production and because operations are so large in scale little attention is given to recovering biologically active organic compounds that may have a much higher unit value than the paper itself. Most of the interesting compounds are in the bark of the tree and during paper processing these go up in smoke when the bark is burnt in boilers to raise power and steam. Some attempts have been made to recover pure lignin for making natural adhesives but the process proved to be uneconomical.

Bark is complex in its chemistry and physical structure, containing literally hundreds of compounds. In a case of the whole being greater than the sum of the parts, all compounds work together in a synergistic way to protect the tree from damage by insects, pests and fungal diseases. Bark can be likened to skin on humans and has similar waterproofing and protective functions. A coniferous tree can repair cuts inflicted on its trunk by marshalling its reserves and exuding resinous compounds to seal off the wound against invaders. It is able to make its very own antiseptic ointment and sticking plaster. The outer, darker, cork layer contains condensed tannins which have a very astringent taste to deter wood-eating insects and bark-browsing animals such as deer. The inner bark, phloem,

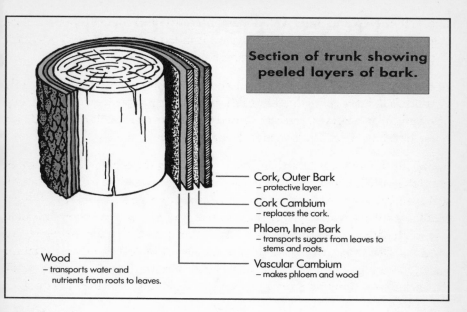

Section of trunk showing peeled layers of bark.

Cork, Outer Bark
– protective layer.

Cork Cambium
– replaces the cork.

Phloem, Inner Bark
– transports sugars from leaves to stems and roots.

Wood
– transports water and nutrients from roots to leaves.

Vascular Cambium
– makes phloem and wood

Figure 1. Section of tree trunk showing peeled layers of bark.

contains more carbohydrates and less tannins which make this a more attractive source of nutrients and medicines for some animals. Goats, sheep, deer, rabbits, and possums instinctively know that a certain amount of new young bark is good for their health and will attack the bark of certain trees, quite often destroying them by ring-barking.

The SAS Handbook of Survival instructs its readers that bark from certain trees is an abundant source of food and nutrients when rendered down by cooking. Some tribes in Africa survive famines by eating the cooked bark from particular trees. One might gain some nutritional and other benefit by chewing raw bark .... but who needs all that fibre?

Bark of a tree is made up of outer and inner bark. The outer bark consists of two layers, the cork and the cork cambium, or cork meristem. The cork is a protective waterproof layer of dead cells which prevents the inner tissues from drying out but still allows these tissues to breathe. This is like the tree's own version of Gortex, a semi-permeable membrane which allows the passage of vapour and gases but not liquid water. The second layer, the cork cambium, is living

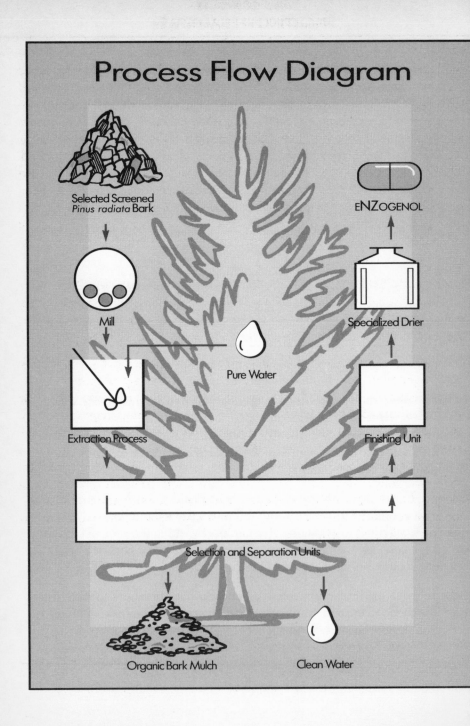

meristematic tissue which replenishes the outer cork as it becomes stretched and torn, worn away or flaked off. The inner bark, called phloem, is a layer of tissue which conducts sugars, manufactured from carbon dioxide and water in the leaves, to the roots and stems where it is stored. Just beneath the phloem is a thin cylindrical sheath of living tissue called the vascular cambium. This is meristematic tissue from which the secondary xylem and phloem are formed. The bark and meristematic tissues from selected parts of the tree trunk are used to make Enzogenol. This ensures that the product includes compounds from the living tissues as well as the dead cork layer. Because oxygen diffuses in from the outside through the bark and meristems, these tissues are rich in the natural antioxidants that play such a vital role in protecting tissues and cells from damage caused by free radicals.

Pinus radiata is the most dominant introduced tree grown in New Zealand for timber and paper production. Over 90% of the total area of all state and private plantations is radiata pine. Who would have believed that the bark from this tree contained compounds with such remarkable nutritive and health giving properties?

Natural, organic Enzogenol is made from carefully selected radiata bark using clean technology which preserves the nutritive and active properties of the compounds in the raw material. These compounds are extracted at the molecular level according to their solubility and size. The process uses latest extraction, membrane separation and water purification technologies. The unique process uses little power and is effective at ensuring Enzogenol is totally sterile. It is a simple, clean, efficient process and produces no waste. The only by-products are a sweet mulch and water. The removed water can be either returned to its source or, after slight purification, reused in the process. A team of scientists and engineers spent three years researching and developing this process. It has now been patented world-wide.

Figure 2 (on opposite page). The Enzogenol production process. Tree bark carefully selected for compliance with certain rigid specifications is extracted with water. The main by-product is a bark residue with wide potential application as a horticultural growing medium and mulch – or as an active ion exchange material for cleaning up heavy metals from industrial effluents.

Assays indicate Enzogenol possesses powerful antioxidant properties compared with many other products. It is a concentrated blend of naturally occurring flavonoids and plant phenols which are capable of protecting the body against attack from free radicals just as they do for the parent tree.

Characterisation and identification of the major constituents of Enzogenol has been taken to great length and so far over thirty components have been positively identified. It is believed there are hundreds altogether. The most active are the ubiquitous proanthocyanidins, as monomers through to oligomers. Also present are some higher molecular weight oligomers which have been shown to have a greater antioxidant activity than the smaller chain oligomeric polyphenols. This is what distinguishes Enzogenol from other products. Research is continuing to identify the unknown compounds so that eventually these will be completely characterised in terms of their specific properties and health benefits in humans. For example it contains cinnamic acid which has recently been shown to have cancer-fighting properties. We strongly suspect the presence of resveratrol and its close cousin astringenin which have been shown to give some protection against cardiac disease. Quercetin, one of the more abundant components, is sometimes prescribed as a natural remedy for the treatment of cardio-vascular problems, such as poor blood circulation. Research on Enzogenol continues. There are many more surprises in store.

References

Hughes, R (1987) *The Fatal Shore: A History of the Transportation of Convicts to Australia.* Collins Harvill, London.

Kinninmonth, J A, Whitehouse, L J (1991) *Properties and Uses of New Zealand Radiata Pine.* Volume 1 Wood Properties. NZ Ministry of Forestry, FRI, Rotorua New Zealand.

Wiseman, J (1986) *The SAS Survival Handbook.* Collins Harvill, London

Chapter 7

Why Enzogenol is an Antioxidant Breakthrough

As we saw in Chapter 4, there are literally thousands of flavonoids, the important dietary compounds in many fruits and vegetables, and there are many different groups of flavonoids with many different biological properties. The molecular selection process used to manufacture Enzogenol captures a mixture from almost every flavonoid group – Enzogenol is an unprecedented encapsulation of the natural defence mechanisms found in many plants, but especially concentrated and diverse in the bark of *Pinus radiata*.

The extraction process used in harvesting this rich mixture plays a key role in Enzogenol's potency.

In the 1950s and 1960s it was taken as gospel that chemical solvents were needed to extract compounds from pine bark. This also applied to other botanicals and, apart from some modifications, those same processes are still in use today. There is a basic problem with this traditional technology. The chemicals extract only parts of the rich mixture and leave behind important compounds that are critical to optimum antioxidant performance. The use of toxic chemicals such as methanol, chloroform, ethyl acetate, methylene chloride and toluene can also leave behind unhealthy residues in the extract. Furthermore, in spite of the toxicity of the solvents used, some resistant micro-organisms can survive to be included in the product.

Enzogenol production, on the other hand, uses only pure water and a molecular selection process. Having developed this breakthrough extraction technique, the scientists then turned to advanced scientific analysis to understand more about what they had produced. They applied the entire analytical arsenal available to them including high performance liquid chromatography (HPLC), gel permeation chromatography (GPC), thin layer chromatography (TLC) and nuclear magnetic resonance (NMR).

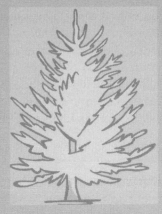

Bark of Pinus radiata

ENZOGENOL

Bark of Pinus radiata	ENZOGENOL
• Monomeric proanthocyanidins	• Monomeric proanthocyanidins
• Oligomeric proanthocyanidins	• Oligomeric proanthocyanidins
• Flavonoids	• Flavonoids
• Organic acids	• Organic acids
• Flavonoid glycosides	• Flavonoid glycosides
• Natural sugars	• Natural sugars
• Esters	• Esters

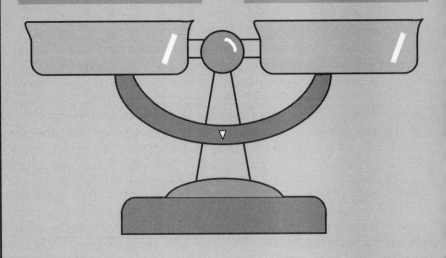

They were genuinely and pleasantly surprised to find that Enzogenol contains more of the higher molecular weight oligomeric proanthocyanidins than any other antioxidant supplement. This key discovery about the molecular composition explains in large part the outstanding results now being reported for Enzogenol, as oligomeric proanthocyanidins are believed to be one of the key groups responsible for enabling the body to fight free radicals. Measurements of the ability of Enzogenol to protect compounds from oxidative damage then confirmed a breakthrough had been achieved.

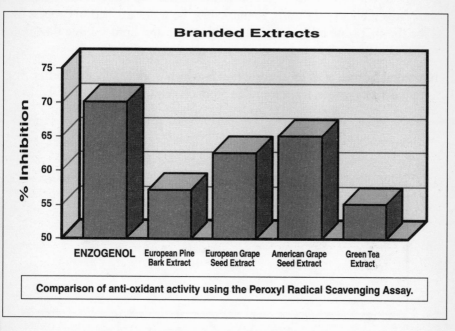

Branded Extracts

Comparison of anti-oxidant activity using the Peroxyl Radical Scavenging Assay.

However, while the presence of higher molecular weight proanthocyanidins explained those unequivocal measurement results to a good extent, the positive feedback the researchers were receiving from early users led them to conclude that other factors were clearly at work as well. They knew that there was another part of the puzzle yet to fit into place if the potency they had unlocked was to be satisfactorily explained.

The answer emerged when they reviewed the extraction technique. The pure water extraction process meant that important natural sugars and organic acids were being included in Enzogenol, just as they are in the tree's natural defence system. Sugars are known to bond with proteins and phenolic molecules to form new compounds. These glyco-proteins or muco-polysacchrides have a number of interesting properties. While the mechanism is not yet well understood, it is likely these bound compounds provide a vehicle for antioxidants to attach to, or even enter, cells – including the critical non-polar parts of the cell.

The sugars may also bind with glycosides and other compounds found in the tree bark to convert the original source molecules into lipid- soluble, in other words fat-soluble, compounds. Remarkably, the water extraction process may be, for the first time ever, harvesting both water and lipid-soluble flavonoids simultaneously.

The natural balance of all those compounds, which work together to form part of the tree's defence system, is not found in products extracted with chemical solvents.

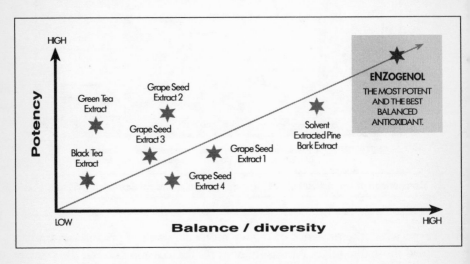

Green and black tea extracts contain mainly monomeric proanthocyanidins, or catechins, and little of the proanthocyanidins such as the important oligomeric groupings, considered essential to a balanced antioxidant. They also contain few of the flavonoid glycosides or esters. While grape seed extracts do contain many of the dimers, trimers and other lower weight proanthocyanidins, they are unfortunately quite variable due to a wide range of raw material sources and extraction methods. Almost all grape seed extracts are produced using powerful solvents, so they suffer from the same shortcomings as other botanicals which are produced with this technology. Grape seed is often incorporated into supplements where low cost, rather than quality or efficacy, is the primary consideration.

Until now solvent-extracted pine bark has been the antioxidant of choice for knowledgeable people. Now they have the opportunity to take a major step forward in the war against free radicals by moving up to Enzogenol.

Chapter 8

Enzogenol: Real Life, Real People

Observations suggest there are two distinct outcomes from taking antioxidants. Readers are now aware of the free radical-destroying effects of antioxidants which result in lesser damage and degeneration. But other effects more immediate effects have been discerned and they are often noticed quickly following the administration of Enzogenol. We call the former *alpha* effects and the latter *beta* effects.

Alpha effects demonstrate themselves in the long term. You may be unaware that the antioxidant is working for you. You have to take it on trust that antioxidants are good for you. They work by mopping up or destroying free radicals. These alpha effects are something like a superannuation scheme. You will not know if you need it until later on in your life. Beta effects, on the other hand, are much more immediately observed. Furthermore, you can feel them doing good to your body and to your activity levels.

In this chapter we relate some of the astounding feedback received from those who have tried Enzogenol. As you will discover, beta effects are more pronounced - because it's what people notice first - but these experiences also hint at longer term alpha benefits coming into play as well.

Some of what you read here may sound fantastic but these reports are true. They have been supplied by real people, and their experiences vary just as their age and health vary. A couple of words of caution are appropriate here. **Should you have any chronic condition you should always consult a health professional.** Enzogenol is not intended as a treatment for a disease or condition – rather it is a supplement to the diet which may well alleviate a shortfall in your body of naturally occurring antioxidants. The benefits of overcoming that shortfall can be dramatic. You do not have to be unwell to derive benefits from Enzogenol.

Establishing the dosage rate that is optimum for you depends on a number of factors. For a healthy fit person who eats a balanced diet, a normal dosage of 50-

150 mg per day will provide a prophylactic amount of antioxidant, conferring the important alpha effect of added protection against the degenerative diseases related to ageing including heart disease, arthritis and cancer.

For specific conditions many have found a higher dosage of 200 to 500 mg per day has given them beta effects and led to health improvement. It is suggested that the daily intake be increased slowly, say over a couple weeks, to higher levels.

In all cases Enzogenol should be taken with main meals.

Judy has been taking Enzogenol for two months starting on a normal dose and increasing it over time. She suffers from lupus and other conditions which for the last two years have seriously disabled her with pain. After taking Enzogenol Judy found pain and stiffness reduced and she was able to decrease her painkiller intake. She can now get out of bed and shower unassisted, and her energy levels are greater than for some years. The pain she does suffer is of "... a much lower grade ..." and she is "... coping much better ...".

Bob, an elderly gentleman, has been on Enzogenol for two months, starting on a low dosage rate and increasing it over time to a high dosage. He had suffered a stroke and a heart attack; he could not get out of bed. He also has a damaged spine. Bob's case was considered critical. After six weeks on Enzogenol he was able to stand. Many of his friends cannot believe how well he looks. His own doctor who had not seen him for a month said he was better than he had seen him in years. Bob can now walk the length of the hospital, is much happier and is feeling great. In fact he is now hoping to leave hospital soon!

Anita has been taking a high dose of Enzogenol for one year. She says it has made a big difference to her life. "It enlightens the soul. It is the difference between night and day – like a cloud had been lifted from me. Everyone comments on how well I look."

Daniel is a youngster with Attention Deficit Disorder. For just under a year, his mother has been giving him a low dose of Enzogenol, off and on. He was a strong-willed and disruptive child who would not listen. He was always on the go and sometimes out of control. Mother said: "He was prescribed medicines by the specialist which caused adverse reactions. Enzogenol quietened him down quite a bit. It mellows him out, and he is not as aggressive which makes things easier for the family. But whenever he stops taking Enzogenol, he reverts back to the way he was."

Wayne suffers from Hodgkinson's disease and is taking a very high dose of Enzogenol. He has been anaemic and at times very tired. Wayne says that since taking Enzogenol he has had a great increase in energy and has been able to do things again. He feels that it has helped him deal with chemotherapy treatment by lifting his energy levels, and he feels he has "... more life ...".

Jim is a long time sufferer of arthritis of the hips, and before taking Enzogenol he used to limp quite severely. Jim says Enzogenol is "... great for inflammation and quietens the pain down". He is on a high dose and takes his capsules twice during the day. The relief effects are felt within about an hour and can last for about 12 hours. It provides a "... slow positive recovery. When you stop taking it the pain and tiredness returns."

Alice has been on a normal dose of Enzogenol for over four months. She has noted an increase in alertness, more energy, and a "definite increase" in motivation and focus. Her skin has improved: " ... it feels a lot smoother ...". Alice says Enzogenol has increased her mental well-being and has a calming effect on her.

Emily is on a normal dose of Enzogenol and describes it as a "natural speed". She says it enhances her mood and gives her a general feeling of well-being. Her personal trainer has noticed a great improvement in her strength and fitness.

Kevin is a busy man and has been taking antioxidant supplements for some time. He describes his body as rather battered from his sports activities – rugby, running, and marathons. He has found that since taking Enzogenol his ailments slightly worsened but then settled down completely. Pains suffered for some time have gone and wound areas have healed. He says he has gone from three and a half years without any major activity to a good level of fitness very quickly, with fellow runners impressed with his rise to fitness. Recently, he damaged his Achilles tendon severely two weeks before a charity marathon. Kevin firmly believes if he were not taking Enzogenol, it would not have healed as well. As it turned out, he was able to run a very long distance over the two days of the event. Interestingly, Kevin is also finding his hair is growing a lot faster.

Gordon has been taking a normal to medium dose of Enzogenol for the last six months. He noted no immediate effect, but over time he realised that he was no longer as tired as he used to be. He has a very physical job. Since on Enzogenol things go more smoothly and easily, and he doesn't feel as worn out.

Lynley has been taking Enzogenol for seven months, starting on a low dose and gradually building up over time. She suffers from rheumatoid arthritis and each year it seems to catch on more joints. Sometimes her body aches all over and when it gets too bad she has had to take strong medication for it. Enzogenol has helped her with this and it seems to "... keep the edge off...". Lynley has noticed the aches and pains return within two to three days after she stops taking Enzogenol. She also has a much improved feeling of well-being. Something else she noticed was that swelling and bruising from a very badly sprained ankle quickly reduced while taking a high dose of Enzogenol. She says "It provided the right environment for healing ... ".

Gail has been taking Enzogenol for four to six months now at a moderate dosage rate. She had been suffering from tennis elbow for about a year before that. There has been "definite improvement" and she says is much more alert.

Una has been taking Enzogenol for nine months. Severe eczema was a frequent result of allergic reactions to cats, feathers and dogs. Since taking Enzogenol, Una has had very few allergic reactions. Indeed, she now has a cat, and can pat it and allow it to rub her face. Friends and family arriving from overseas could not believe the improvement. She says everyone comments on how much younger and more healthy she looks. Una can now wear make-up, something she could not do regularly before. She can now swim without fear of her skin reacting to the chlorine. Una had severe chicken pox some months ago and was concerned about possible scarring, but her skin cleared up extremely well. She says she is now stronger physically, has less colds and flu, sleeps better and enjoys a general improvement in immunity. "I haven't looked back since taking Enzogenol."

Lynne, a sufferer of a chronic condition causing much pain and discomfort, has been on a high dose of Enzogenol for six months after being on other antioxidant supplements previously. She says she gradually started to feel better. Lynne was having a lot of trouble moving around and doctors were advising a partial amputation of a leg, which she refused. She is now comfortably moving around, her morphine intake has decreased and she is eating better. She has also had improved healing of the ulcers and sores that she gets due to her condition. Lynne is very positive about Enzogenol and says she will not stop taking it.

Nedra, an arthritis sufferer, has been taking Enzogenol for nine months. She has increased her dosage from normal to a high one, and feels she is a long way ahead of where she was six months before. She does not need her regular Vitamin B12 shots as often as previously, is experiencing a gradually increasing feeling of well-being, is finding she is coping with things a lot better and is enjoying better quality sleep on a more regular basis. She also says she is suffering less arthritic pain in her wrists and arms. She thinks Enzogenol helps with healing as well, saying a twisted ankle recovered more quickly than she would have expected. Nedra's husband says she has improved immensely, calling Enzogenol "... a godsend".

Rob has been taking Enzogenol for 18 months now. While he considers himself to be a regular user, the main thing he has noticed is that when he takes Enzogenol he doesn't suffer from cold sores, but they become a problem again when he stops taking it.

Alex has been taking Enzogenol regularly for one year. He used to suffer intense migraines, with associated vomiting and stomach queasiness, at frequent intervals and needed strong medication to ease them. Certain combinations of foods caused an upset stomach. Since taking Enzogenol, he has been dramatically different – the migraines have gone, he no longer suffers from nausea or indigestion, now eats foods in any combination and has no "off colour" days. Occasional slight headaches are quickly dispelled by extra capsules, in place of medication. Alex finds he has more energy reserves and has established this is related to Enzogenol dose levels. He takes extra capsules to eradicate fatigue and prevent jet lag on long flights. He has also noticed improvement in his skin condition.

Julian is not a regular taker of Enzogenol, but takes it when he is feeling tired and needs an energy boost. He also takes it when he is feeling 'fluey' and says it is very good for a hangover!

Chapter 9

A Recipe for Healthy Living
by Dr Kelvin Duncan

In this book we have tried to indicate what modern science can tell us about the role of free radicals in disease, ageing and degeneration of the human body. As we have indicated, there are a great many things we know about the activity of free radicals, and more is being learned almost literally every day. But in free radical research so much is still the subject of suspicion, conjecture and estimation. So what we say is not the final word on the subject. We have, however, made an honest attempt to acquaint you with a reasonable summary of current knowledge and thinking about the vital role antioxidants play in human health.

We know that oxidising free radicals exist and that they wreak havoc in our bodies that is often irreversible. Unfortunately, the life of free radicals is in most cases too unbelievably brief, and all cases too microscopic, to observe. Controlled laboratory experiments to test many of the suppositions presented in this book are impossible.

We know that free radical activity can be curbed by antioxidants. We know that plants produce antioxidants in great quantity and diversity for the benefit of themselves and of the animals that eat them. We know the human body produces antioxidants, but not enough of them. There is a great deal of probability that supplementing your diet with concentrated antioxidants will help protect your body against the diseases mentioned throughout this book, but there is by no means certainty that this is the case. The scientists and the technologists will continue their work and, in time, a great deal more will be known than is so today.

So let us repeat our recipe for healthy living. If we are right then you should:

Consult a medical practitioner in all cases where you have an obvious illness.

Consult a medical practitioner for regular (yearly) check-ups. This is especially important for men. From one bloke to another - don't be too macho and think you are invincible and do not need to go to a doctor. Plenty of younger men in the graveyard would sorrowfully attest to the foolishness of that attitude!

Enjoy eating plenty of green vegetables and fruits in the least processed form possible for you.

Follow sensible dietary advice. Cut down on fatty foods, especially those that are known to raise blood cholesterol levels.

Enjoy regular exercise appropriate to your age and condition. If your current exercise regime is not enjoyable, then change it. You are doing the wrong exercise.

Learn to listen to your body. You have a great number of powerful feedback mechanisms that are designed to tell you when something is going wrong. Listen to and respect them. Help your body heal itself. Humans are wonderfully endowed with regenerative capacities that can heal and repair if given the chance. Use them.

Avoid undue exposure to damaging radiation, such as UV and sunlight - cover up when outside by using clothing or an effective sunblock.

Enjoy regular and plentiful sleep.

Avoid stress at work or in your personal life. If your life is in a mess then seek professional help. You may not be able to sort yourself out alone and great damage can be done by the stress that you are experiencing.

Enjoy all things in moderation.

Take antioxidant supplements, such as Enzogenol, in a dose appropriate for your size and level of activity. Let your body tell you the appropriate dosage.

Your body is different from everyone else's. The way it responds to foods, drinks and medicinal drugs will often be different, usually only slightly but in some cases significantly, from reactions experienced by other people. How your body will respond to Enzogenol, then, is hard to predict. Almost all who have taken courses report a heightened feeling of well-being and differing degrees of alleviation of ailments they have been suffering. Some have noted other changes too – mor e energy, less depression, better sleep. A parallel of changes observed in the long-living mice has also been experienced by some: faster hair growth. We can postulate that this is a sign of a healthier body, but we really do not know. A strong hint that Enzogenol is the agent of these changes lies in many reports that when dosage is discontinued, the beneficial effects experienced have dissipated. To date, no person taking Enzogenol has reported any negative side effects.

One thing of which you can be confident, however, is that diet supplementation with antioxidants is well beyond what is commonly referred to as 'fringe' medicine. Aspirin was regarded as fringe thinking when it was first introduced. How many would see it that way today? So it is with antioxidants. The mounting evidence is far too weighty, too credible, for any of us to state that taking antioxidants is a pointless exercise. The fact that the astounding propositions in this book are being advanced by highly regarded scientists working in our most prominent universities should alone transmit that we are on the brink of a very exciting medical breakthrough.

We can also be assured that, in Enzogenol, we have for the first time a very safe antioxidant product that reproduces nature's own free radical defence mechanism as precisely as present technology will allow. In Enzogenol, we have exactly the same free radical-fighting force as millions of years of evolution have devised for the humble pine tree.

As I write this I can almost hear a faint echo of what my grandmother told me when I was a child about how to live a healthy and productive life. So what we say repeats in large measure the wisdom of the ages as told me by my Gran. We do not deny this immense collection of wisdom. It has been proven by millions. Indeed, we believe have added to it.

Good health!

Further Reading

Afanasíev, I G, Dorozhko, A I, Brodskii, A V, Kostyuk, A, Potapovitch, A I, (1989) "Chelating and Free Radical Scavenging Mechanisms of Inhibitory Action of Rutin and Quercetin in Lipid Peroxidation." *Biochemical Pharmacology*, Vol 38.

Ames, B N, Shigenaga, M K, and Hagen, T M (1993) "Oxidants, Antioxidants, and the Degenerative Diseases of Aging." *Proc. Natl. Acad. Sci.*, Vol 90.

Block, G, Langseth, L. (1994) "Antioxidant Vitamins and Disease Prevention." *Food Technology*, July.

Block, G, Patterson, B, Subar, A. (1992) "Fruit, Vegetables and Cancer Prevention: A Review of the Epidemiological Evidence." *Nutrition and Cancer*, Vol 18, No 1.

Block, G. (1992) "The Data Support a Role for Antioxidants in Reducing Cancer Risk." *Nutrition Reviews*, Vol 50, No 7.

Bors, W, Heller, W, Michel, C and Saran, M. (1990) "Flavonoids as Antioxidants: Determination of Radical-Scavenging Efficiencies." *Methods in Enzymology*, Vol 186.

Cadenas, E, Packer, L, eds (1996) *Handbook of Antioxidants*. Marcel Dekker, Inc, New York.

Cao, G, Sofic, E, Prior, R L.(1997) "Antioxidant and Prooxidant Behaviour of Flavonoids: Structure-Activity Relationships." *Free Radical Biology & Medicine*, Vol 22, No 5.

Cerruti, P A. (1976) "Oxy-radicals and Cancer." *Lancet*, Vol 344.

Cheeseman K H, Slater, T F, (1993) "An Introduction to Free Radical Biochemistry." *British Medical Bulletin*, Vol 49.

Chen, C.M., and Pan, J.K. (1991) "Effects of Extraction on Yields and Characteristics of Bark Extracts." *Holzforshung*, Vol 45.

Cody, V, Middleton, E, Harborne, JB, eds (1986) *Plant Flavonoids in Biology and Medicine: Biochemical, Pharmacological, and Structure-Activity Relationships*. Alan R. Liss, New York.

Cook, N C, Samman, S. (1996) "Flavonoids - Chemistry, Metabolism, Cardioprotective Effects and Dietary Sources." *J. Nutr. Biochem.*, Vol 7.

Cross, C E. (1987) "Proceedings of the Davis Conference: Oxygen Radicals and Human Disease." *Annals of Internal Medicine*. Vol 107.

Da Silva Emim, J A., Oliveira, A B., and Lapa, A J. (1994) "Pharmacological Evaluation of the Anti-inflammatory Activity of a Citrus Bioflavonoid, Hesperidin, and the Isoflavonoids, Duratin and Claussequinone, in Rats and Mice." *J. Pharm. Pharmacol.*, Vol 46.

Das, D K. (1994) "Naturally occurring Flavonoids: Structure, Chemistry, and High-Performance

Liquid Chromatography Methods for Separation and Characterisation." *Methods of Enzymology*, Vol 234.

De Whalley, C V, Rankin, S M, Hoult, R S, Jessup, W, Leake, D S. (1990) "Flavonoids Inhibit the Oxidative Modification of Low Density Lipoproteins by Macrophages." *Biochemical Pharmacology*, Vol 39, No 11.

Dey PM, Harborne, JB, eds (1989) "Methods in Plant Biochemistry." Vol 1. *Plant Phenolics*, Academic Press, London.

Fishman, R H B. (1994) "Antioxidants and Phytotherapy." Lancet, Vol 344.

Formica, J V and Regelson, W. (1995) "Review of the Biology of Quercetin and Related Bioflavonoids." *Fd Chem. Toxic.*, Vol 33, No 12.

Gali, H U, Perchellet, E M, Gao, X M, Karchesy, J J, Perchellet, J P. (1994) "Comparison of the Inhibitory Effects of Monomeric, Dimeric, and Trimeric Procyanidins on the Biochemical Markers of Skin Tumour Promotion in Mouse Epidermis *in vivo*." *Plant Med.*, Vol 60.

Grisham, M B. (1994) "Oxidants and Free Radicals in Inflammatory Bowel Disease." *Lancet*, Vol 344.

Halliwell, B, Gutteridge, J M C and Cross, C E. (1992) "Free Radicals, Antioxidants, and Human Disease: Where Are We Now?" J Lab Clin Med, Vol 119, No 6.

Halliwell, B, Gutteridge, JMC (1989) *Free Radicals in Biology and Medicine*, 2nd Edition, Claredon Press, Oxford.

Halliwell, B. (1994) "Free Radicals, Anti-Oxidants, and Human Disease: Curiosity, Cause, Or Consequence?" *Lancet*, Vol 344.

Halliwell, B. (1995) "Oxidation of Low-density lipoproteins: Questions of Initiation, Propagation, and the Effect of Antioxidants." *Am J Clin Nutr.*, Vol 61.

Harborne, JB, ed (1988) *The Flavonoids - Advances in Research Since 1980*. Chapman and Hall, London.

Harborne, JB, ed (1994) *The Flavonoids - Advances in Research since 1986*. Academic Press, London.

Harborne, JB, Mabry TJ, Mabry H, eds (1975) *The Flavonoids*. Chapman and Hall, London.

Herrmann, K (1976) "Flavonols and Flavones in Food Plants: a Review. *J. Fd. Technol.* Vol 11.

Herrmann, K (1988) "On the Occurrence of Flavonol and Flavone Glycosides in Vegetables." *Ubersichtsbericht.* Vol 186.

Herrmann, K (1989) "Occurrence and Content of Hydroxycinnamic and Hydroxybenzoic Acid Compounds in Foods." *Critical Reviews in Food Science and Nutrition.* Vol 28, Issue 4.

Hertog, M G L, Feskens E J M, Hollman P C H, Katan M B, Kromhout, D. (1993) "Dietary Antioxidant Flavonoids and Risk of Coronary Heart Disease: The Zutphen Elderly Study." *Lancet,* Vol 342.

Hertog, M G L, Hollman P C H, Katan M B and Kromhout, D. (1993) "Intake of Potentially Anticarcinogenic Flavonoids and Their Determinants in Adults in The Netherlands." *Nutrition and Cancer,* Vol 20, No 1.

Hertog, M G L, Hollman P C H, Katan M B. (1992) "Content of Potentially Anticarcinogenic Flavonoids of 28 Vegetables and 9 Fruits Commonly Consumed in The Netherlands." *J Agric Food Chem,* Vol 40.

Hertog, M G L, Hollman P C H. (1996) "Potential Health Effects of the Dietary Flavonol Quercetin." *European Journal of Clinical Nutrition,* Vol 50.

Hertog, M G L, Kromhout, D, Aravanis, C, Blackburn, H, Buzina, R, et al,. (1995) "Flavonoid Intake and Long-term Risk of Coronary Heart Disease and Cancer in the Seven Countries Study." *Arch Intern Med,* Vol 155.

Hertog, M G L. (1996) "Epidemiological Evidence on Potential Health Properties of Flavonoids." *Proceedings of the Nutrition Society,* Vol 55.

Hollman, P C H, Katan, M B. (1997) "Absorption , Metabolism and Health Effects of Dietary Flavonoids in Man." *Biomed & Pharmacother,* Vol 51.

Hollman, P C H., Gaag, M V D., Mengelers, M J B., van Trup, J M P., de Vries, J H M., Katan, M B. (1996) "Absorption and Disposition Kinetics of the Dietary Antioxidant Quercetin in Man." *Free Radical Biology and Medicine,* Vol 21, No 5.

Huang, M-T, Ho, C-H, Lee, CY eds (1992) *Phenolic Compounds in Food and Their Effects on Health I and II.* American Chemical Society, Washington, DC.

Husain, S R, Cillard, J, Cillard, P (1987) "Hydroxyl Radical Scavenging Activity of Flavonoids." *Phytochemistry,* Vol 26, No 9.

Jacques, P F, Chylack, L T (1991) "Epidemiological Evidence of a Role for the Antioxidant Vitamins and Carotenoids in Cataract Prevention." *Am J Clin Nutr,* Vol 53.

Jenner, P. (1994) "Oxidative Damage in Neuerodegenerative Disease." *Lancet, Vol 344.*

Kandaswami, C, Middleton, E. (1994) "Free Radical Scavenging and Antioxidant Activity of Plant Flavonoids." From *Free Radicals in Diagnostic Medicine,* Edited by D Armstrong, Plenum Press New York.

Keli, S O, Hertog M G L, Feskens E J M, Kromhout D. (1996) "Dietary Flavonoids, Antioxidant Vitamins, and Incidence of Stroke." *Arch. Intern. Med,* Vol 156.

Kininmonth. JA, Whitehouse, LJ eds (1991) *Properties and Uses of New Zealand Radiata Pine, Volume 1, - Wood Properties*. NZ Ministry of Forestry, Forest Research Institute, Rotorua, New Zealand.

Knekt, P, Jarvinen, R, Reunanen, A, Maatela. (1996) "Flavonoid Intake and Coronary Mortality in Finland: a Cohort Study." *BMJ, Vol 312*.

Kuhnau, J. (1976) "The Flavonoids. A Class of Semi-Essential Food Components: Their Role in Human Nutrition." *Wld Rev. Nutr Diet.*, Vol 24.

Lei, L, Hudgins, W R, Shack, S, Yin M Q, Samid, D., (1995) "Cinnamic Acid: A Natural Product with Potential Use in Cancer Intervention." *Int. J. Cancer*, Vol 62.

Lotito, S B, and Fraga, C G. (1998) "(U)-Catechin Prevents Human Plasma Oxidation." *Free Radical Biology & Medicine*, Vol 24, No 3.

Markham, K.R. and Porter, L.J. (1973) "Extractives of *Pinus radiata* Bark. 1. Phenolic Components." *New Zealand Journal of Science*, Vol 16.

Markham, KR, (1982) *Techniques in Flavonoid Identification*. Academic Press, London.

Middleton, E. (1996) "Biological Properties of Plant Flavonoids: An Overview." *International Journal of Pharmacognosy*, Vol 34, No 5.

Miller, N J, Rice-Evans C A. (1996) "Spectrophotometric Determination of Antioxidant Activity." *Redox Report*, Vol 2, No 3.

Packer, L, (1993) Letter to the Editor: "Health Effects of Nutritional Antioxidants." *Free Radical Biology & Medicine*, Vol 15.

Porter, L.J. (1974) "Extractives of Pinus radiata bark. 2. Procyanidin constituents." *New Zealand Journal of Science*, Vol 17.

Porter, L.J. and Foo, L.P. (1980) "Differences in Condensed Tannin Structures in Pine Bark as a Function of Tree Age." Taken from The Pulping and Papermaking Properties of Radiata Pine Corewood (Juvenile Wood) *FRI Symposium* No 23.

Pryor, W A, Cornicelli J A, Devall, L J, Tait, B, Trivedi, B K, Witiak, D T and Wu, M.(1993) "A Rapid Screening Test to Determine the Antioxidant Potencies of Natural and Synthetic Antioxidants." *J. Org. Chem.*, Vol 58, No 13.

Rice-Evans, C, (1995) "Plant Polyphenols: Free Radical Scavengers or Chain-breaking Antioxidants?" *Biochem. Soc. Symp*, Vol 61.

Rice-Evans, C. A., Miller, N. J., Bolwell, P. G., Bramley, P. M., Pridham, J. B. (1995) "The Relative Antioxidant Activities of Plant-Derived Polyphenolic Flavonoids." *Free Rad Res*, Vol 22, No 4.

Rice-Evans, C. A., Miller, N. J., Paganda, G. (1996) "Structure-Antioxidant Activity Relationships of Flavonoids and Phenolic Acids." *Free Radical Biology & Medicine*, Vol 20, No 7.

Rice-Evans, CA, Packer, L, eds (1998) *Flavonoids in Health and Disease*. Marcel Dekker, Inc New York.

Robak, J, Gryglewski, R J. (1988) "Flavonoids are Scavengers of Superoxide Anions." *Biochemical Pharmacology*, Vol 37, No 5.

Scalbert, A., Monties, B., and Janin, G. (1989) "Tannins in Wood: Comparison of Different Estimation Methods." *J Agric. Food Chem.*, Vol 37.

Stavric, B. (1994) "Role of Chemopreventers in Human Diet." *Clinical Biochemistry*, Vol 27, No 5.

Tewes, F J, Koo, L C, Meisgen, T J, Rylander R. (1990) "Lung Cancer Risk and Mutagenicity of Tea." *Environmental Research*, Vol 52.

van Acker, S A B E, van den Berg D, Tromp, M N J L, Griffioen, D H, van Bennekom, van der Vijgh and Bast, A. (1996) "Structural Aspects of Antioxidant Activity of Flavonoids." *Free Radical Biology & Medicine*, Vol 20, No 3.

Vile, G F, Tyrell, R M. (1995) "UVA Radiation-Induced Oxidative Damage to Lipids and Proteins *in vitro* and in Human Skin Fibroblasts is Dependent on Iron and Singlet Oxygen." *Free Radical Biology and Medicine*, Vol 18, No 4.

Williams, V.M., Porter, L.J., and Hemingway, R.W. (1983) "Molecular Weight Profiles of Proanthocyanidin Polymers." *Phytochemistry*, Vol 22, No 2.

Winterbourn, C C., (1995) "Nutritional Antioxidants: Their Role in Disease Prevention." *New Zealand Medical Journal*, Vol 108 No 1011.

Witzum, J L, (1994) "The Oxidation Hypothesis of Atherosclerosis." *Lancet*, Vol 344.

Yazaki, Y. (1985) "Extraction of Polyphenols from *Pinus radiata* Bark." *Holzforshung*, Vol 39.

Yazaki, Y. (1987) "Solubility of Extracts from *Pinus radiata* Bark" *Holzforshung*, Vol 41.

Yazaki, Y. and Aung, T,. (1988) "Polyphenolic Extractives of *Pinus radiata* Bark." *Holzforshung*, Vol 31.

Yazaki, Y. and Hillis, W.E. (1977) "Polyphenolic Extractives of *Pinus radiata* Bark." *Holzforshung*, Vol 31.

Yazaki, Y. and Hillis, W.E. (1980) "Molecular Size Distribution of Radiata Pine Bark Extracts and its Effect on Properties." *Holzforshung*, Vol 34.

Yu, C L, and Swaminathan, B. (1987) "Mutagenicity of Proanthocyanidins." *Fd Chem. Toxic.*, Vol 25, No 2.

Yuting, C, Rongliang, Z, Zhongjian, J, Yong, J. (1990) "Flavonoids as Superoxide Scavengers and Antioxidants." *Free Radical Biology & Medicine*, Vol 9.